Androgens in Women: Too Much, Too Little, Just Right

Editor

MARGARET E. WIERMAN

ENDOCRINOLOGY AND METABOLISM CLINICS OF NORTH AMERICA

www.endo.theclinics.com

Consulting Editor
ADRIANA G. IOACHIMESCU

March 2021 • Volume 50 • Number 1

ELSEVIER

1600 John F. Kennedy Boulevard • Suite 1800 • Philadelphia, Pennsylvania, 19103-2899

http://www.theclinics.com

ENDOCRINOLOGY AND METABOLISM CLINICS OF NORTH AMERICA Volume 50, Number 1
March 2021 ISSN 0889-8529, ISBN 13: 978-0-323-77736-0

Editor: Katerina Heidhausen
Developmental Editor: Nicole Congleton

Endocrinology and Metabolism Clinics of North America (ISSN 0889-8529) is published quarterly by Elsevier Inc., 360 Park Avenue South, New York, NY 10010-1710. Months of issue are March, June, September, and December. Periodicals postage paid at New York, NY and additional mailing offices. Subscription prices are USD 383.00 per year for US individuals, USD 1037.00 per year for US institutions, USD 100.00 per year for US students and residents, USD 454.00 per year for Canadian individuals, USD 1089.00 per year for Canadian institutions, USD 497.00 per year for international individuals, USD 1089.00 per year for international institutions, USD 100.00 per year for Canadian students/residents, and USD 245.00 per year for international students/residents. To receive student/resident rate, orders must be accompanied by name of affiliated institution, date of term, and the signature of program/residency coordinator on institution letterhead. Orders will be billed at individual rate until proof of status is received. Foreign air speed delivery is included in all *Clinics* subscription prices. All prices are subject to change without notice. **POSTMASTER:** Send address changes to *Endocrinology and Metabolism Clinics of North America*, Elsevier Health Sciences Division, Subscription Customer Service, 3251 Riverport Lane, Maryland Heights, MO 63043. **Customer Service: Telephone: 1-800-654-2452** (U.S. and Canada); **1-314-447-8871** (outside U.S. and Canada). **Fax: 1-314-447-8029. E-mail: journalscustomerservice-u-sa@elsevier.com (for print support); journalsonlinesupport-usa@elsevier.com (for online support).**

Reprints. For copies of 100 or more, of articles in this publication, please contact the Commercial Rights Department, Elsevier Inc., 360 Park Avenue South, New York, NY 10010-1710; phone: +1-212-633-3874; fax: +1-212-633-3820; E-mail: reprints@elsevier.com.

Endocrinology and Metabolism Clinics of North America is covered in *MEDLINE/PubMed (Index Medicus), EMBASE/Excerpta Medica, Current Contents/Clinical Medicine, Current Contents/Life Sciences, Science Citation Index, ISI/BIOMED, BIOSIS,* and *Chemical Abstracts*.

Contributors

CONSULTING EDITOR

ADRIANA G. IOACHIMESCU, MD, PhD, FACE
Professor, Departments of Medicine, Endocrinology and Metabolism, and Neurosurgery, Emory University, Emory University School of Medicine, Atlanta, Georgia, USA

EDITOR

MARGARET E. WIERMAN, MD
Division of Endocrinology, Diabetes, and Metabolism, Professor in Medicine, Integrative Physiology, Director, Pituitary Adrenal and Neuroendocrine Tumor Program, Chief of Endocrinology, Rocky Mountain Regional VA Medical Center, University of Colorado Anschutz Medical Campus, University of Colorado School of Medicine, Aurora, Colorado, USA

AUTHORS

LINDA A. BARBOUR, MD, MSPH
Departments of Medicine and Obstetrics and Gynecology, University of Colorado Anschutz Medical Campus, Aurora, Colorado, USA

ROSEMARY BASSON, MD, FRCP(UK)
Clinical Professor, Department of Psychiatry, University of British Columbia, Vancouver, British Columbia, Canada

ISABELLA BLACKMAN, BA
Department of Obstetrics and Gynecology, Division of Midlife Health, Midlife Health Center, University of Virginia Health System, Charlottesville, Virginia, USA

CHRISTINE M. BURT SOLORZANO, MD
Associate Professor of Pediatrics, Center for Research in Reproduction, Department of Pediatrics, Division of Endocrinology and Metabolism, University of Virginia School of Medicine, University of Virginia Health, Charlottesville, Virginia, USA

SYDNEY CHANG, MD
Department of Obstetrics and Gynecology, Division of Reproductive Endocrinology, Donald and Barbara Zucker School of Medicine at Hofstra/Northwell, New York, New York, USA

EDWARD ALEXANDER CONNER, MD
Department of Obstetrics and Gynecology, Division of Midlife Health, Midlife Health Center, University of Virginia Health System, Charlottesville, Virginia, USA

LAURA G. COONEY, MD
Department of Obstetrics and Gynecology, University of Wisconsin, Generations Fertility Care, Middleton, Wisconsin, USA

SUSAN R. DAVIS, MBBS, FRACP, PhD, FAHMS
Professor, Women's Health Research Program, School of Public Health and Preventive Medicine, Monash University, Melbourne, Victoria, Australia

ANUJA DOKRAS, MD, PhD
Department of Obstetrics and Gynecology, University of Pennsylvania, Penn Fertility Care, Philadelphia, Pennsylvania, USA

ANDREA DUNAIF, MD
Professor of Medicine, Endocrinology, Diabetes and Bone Disease, Icahn School of Medicine at Mount Sinai, Chief of the Hilda and J. Lester Gabrilove Division of Endocrinology, Diabetes and Bone Disease, New York, New York, USA

SMITA JHA, MD
Assistant Research Physician, Section on Congenital Disorders, National Institutes of Health Clinical Center, Metabolic Diseases Branch, National Institutes of Diabetes and Digestive and Kidney Diseases, Bethesda, Maryland, USA

ANDREW M. KAUNITZ, MD, NCMP
University of Florida College of Medicine Jacksonville, UF Health Women's Specialists, Jacksonville, Florida, USA

CHRISTOPHER R. McCARTNEY, MD
Professor of Medicine, Center for Research in Reproduction, Department of Medicine, Division of Endocrinology and Metabolism, University of Virginia School of Medicine, University of Virginia Health, Charlottesville, Virginia, USA

JOANN V. PINKERTON, MD, NCMP
Professor of Obstetrics and Gynecology, Division Director of Midlife Health, Executive Director Emeritus, The North American Menopause Society, Department of Obstetrics and Gynecology, Division of Midlife Health, Midlife Health Center, University of Virginia Health System, Charlottesville, Virginia, USA

MICOL S. ROTHMAN, MD
Professor, Division of Endocrinology, Metabolism and Diabetes, Department of Medicine, University of Colorado Anschutz Medical Campus, Aurora, Colorado, USA

JOHN S. RUSHING, MD
Department of Obstetrics and Gynecology, University of Colorado, Aurora, Colorado, USA

NANETTE SANTORO, MD
Chair, Department of Obstetrics and Gynecology, University of Colorado, Aurora, Colorado, USA

ADINA F. TURCU, MD, MS
Assistant Professor, Division of Metabolism, Endocrinology and Diabetes, University of Michigan, Ann Arbor, Michigan, USA

AMY M. VALENT, DO
Department of Obstetrics and Gynecology, Oregon Health & Science University, Portland, Oregon, USA

CORRINE K. WELT, MD
George Cartwright Endowed Chair in Internal Medicine, Professor of Internal Medicine, Chief, Division of Endocrinology, Metabolism and Diabetes, University of Utah School of Medicine, Salt Lake City, Utah, USA

MARGARET E. WIERMAN, MD
Division of Endocrinology, Diabetes, and Metabolism, Professor in Medicine, Integrative Physiology, Director, Pituitary Adrenal and Neuroendocrine Tumor Program, Chief of Endocrinology, Rocky Mountain Regional VA Medical Center, University of Colorado Anschutz Medical Campus, University of Colorado School of Medicine, Aurora, Colorado, USA

ADNIN ZAMAN, MD
Clinical/Research Fellow, Division of Endocrinology, Metabolism and Diabetes, Department of Medicine, University of Colorado Anschutz Medical Campus, Aurora, Colorado, USA

Contents

> Hyperandrogenic anovulation refers to the constellation of disorders that present in women with irregular menses, hirsutism and/or acne across the lifespan. Understanding the clinical signs and symptoms of each diagnosis in the differential and laboratory testing to confirm or exclude a diagnosis allows a clinician to appropriately counsel and treat the patient.

> Current diagnostic criteria for polycystic ovary syndrome (PCOS) are based on expert opinion. This article reviews the rationale for and the limitations of these criteria as well as which criteria to use and when. The insights provided into PCOS pathogenesis by modern genetic analyses and the promise of objective data mining approaches for biologically relevant disease classification are discussed.

> The pathophysiology of symptomatic polycystic ovary syndrome (PCOS) often unfolds across puberty, but the ontogeny of PCOS is difficult to study because, in general, its pathophysiology is well entrenched before the diagnosis can be confirmed. However, the study of high-risk groups (daughters of women with PCOS, girls with premature pubarche, and girls with obesity) can offer insight in this regard. Available data support the hypothesis that the pubertal development of PCOS involves various combinations of genetic predisposition, intrauterine programming, hyperinsulinism, and numerous other abnormalities that provoke reproductive symptoms (eg, hyperandrogenism, ovulatory dysfunction) in response to the pubertal increase in gonadotropin secretion.

> The triad of hirsutism, amenorrhea, and enlarged polycystic ovaries first was described in 1935 and later become known as polycystic ovarian syndrome (PCOS). Women with PCOS are more likely to have cardiometabolic

challenges that also have an indirect relationship to their fertility and fertility outcomes. Despite these challenges, their fertile life span appears to be longer. Ovulation induction is considered first-line management of infertility in women with PCOS, with letrozole superior to clomiphene. Women with PCOS undergoing in vitro fertilization are high risk for ovarian hyperstimulation syndrome but also have a higher live birth rate compared with controls.

Management of Women with Polycystic Ovary Syndrome During Pregnancy   57

Amy M. Valent and Linda A. Barbour

Polycystic ovary syndrome (PCOS) is the most common endocrinopathy among reproductive age women and is associated with subfertility and adverse perinatal outcomes, which may include early pregnancy loss, gestational diabetes mellitus, hypertensive spectrum disorder, preterm birth, fetal growth disorders, and cesarean deliveries. The phenotypic heterogeneity, different diagnostic criteria, and PCOS-related conditions that women enter pregnancy with have limited evidenced-based studies and guidelines to reduce pregnancy complications among this high-risk population. This review summarizes the available evidence on the approach and management of women with PCOS preconception, prenatal, and postpartum.

Genetics of Polycystic Ovary Syndrome: What is New?   71

Corrine K. Welt

Polycystic ovary syndrome (PCOS) is a complex genetic disorder with many genetic loci contributing small risk. Large genome-wide association studies identified 21 genetic risk loci for PCOS in European and Han Chinese women. The genetic architecture is similar across PCOS diagnostic categories. The next wave of analysis will incorporate large genotyped datasets linked to medical records, increasing numbers and ethnic subsets. The resulting genetic risk loci can then be used to create robust genetic risk scores enhanced with clinical information, environment and lifestyle data for a precision medicine approach to PCOS diagnosis and treatment.

Cardiometabolic Risk in Polycystic Ovary Syndrome: Current Guidelines   83

Laura G. Cooney and Anuja Dokras

Polycystic ovary syndrome is a common endocrine disorder in reproductive-aged women and is associated with an increased risk of metabolic abnormalities, including obesity, impaired glucose tolerance, diabetes, dyslipidemia, metabolic syndrome, venous thromboembolism, and subclinical atherosclerosis. Clinicians and patients alike need to be aware of these increased risks as well as new international guidelines that recommend frequent screening and active management of metabolic abnormalities. Given that the data on risk of cardiovascular events, such as myocardial infarction and stroke, in women with PCOS is mixed, future large-scale, longitudinal studies are needed to clarify these potential risks.

Congenital adrenal hyperplasia encompasses a group of autosomal recessive defects in cortisol biosynthesis, and 21-hydroxylase deficiency accounts for 95% of such cases. Non-classic 21-hydroxylase deficiency is due to partial enzymatic defects, which present with normal cortisol synthesis, but excessive production of adrenal androgens, including 11-oxygenated androgens. Non-classic 21-hydroxylase deficiency is relatively common, and its phenotype resembles closely that of polycystic ovary syndrome. This review focuses primarily on non-classic 21-hydroxylase deficiency, its clinical features, diagnosis, and management.

ENDOCRINOLOGY AND METABOLISM CLINICS OF NORTH AMERICA

Foreword

Androgens in Women: Too Much, Too Little, Just Right

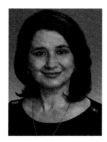

Adriana G. Ioachimescu, MD, PhD, FACE
Consulting Editor

It is my great pleasure to announce the new issue of the *Endocrinology and Metabolism Clinics of North America* dedicated to the role and pathologic condition of androgen hormones in women. The guest editor is Dr Margaret E. Wierman, Professor of Medicine, Obstetrics, and Gynecology at the University of Colorado School of Medicine. Dr Wierman is a leader in the field and has authored multiple publications on the physiology of hormone secretion during the menstrual cycle, pathophysiologic pathways of hypogonadism, sexual dysfunction, androgen excess, and androgen use in women. Dr Wierman has also served as the Chair of the Endocrine Society Guidelines committee on the therapeutic use of androgens in women.

In recent years, progress has been made regarding measuring androgen levels and defining the hyperandrogenic pathologic condition in women. This issue provides updates regarding patient evaluation and differential diagnosis among the possible causes of hyperandrogenism in women. A common diagnosis is polycystic ovarian syndrome, which is addressed by several articles focused on its genetic subtypes, manifestations in adolescence, fertility implications, preconception and pregnancy care, variable clinical phenotype, as well as metabolic and cardiovascular comorbidities. Less frequent causes of hyperandrogenism are also addressed, including the nonclassical adrenal hyperplasia, tumoral hyperandrogenism, and hyperthecosis. An emerging topic is the role of androgens in sexual function and dysfunction in women. This is thoughtfully reviewed along with the decision of whether to attempt a trial of testosterone therapy in postmenopausal women with hypoactive sexual desire disorder and balance potential benefits with adverse effects.

I hope you will find this issue of the *Endocrinology and Metabolism Clinics of North America* useful for your practice for new research projects. I thank Dr Wierman for guest-editing this important collection of articles and the authors for their tremendous

Endocrinol Metab Clin N Am 50 (2021) xiii–xiv
https://doi.org/10.1016/j.ecl.2020.12.005
0889-8529/21/© 2020 Published by Elsevier Inc.

contributions. I also would like to recognize the Elsevier editorial staff, who supported the authors and editors at every step.

Adriana G. Ioachimescu, MD, PhD, FACE
Emory University School of Medicine
1365 B Clifton Road, Northeast, B6209
Atlanta, GA 30322, USA

E-mail address:
aioachi@emory.edu

Preface

Why Focus on Androgens in Women?

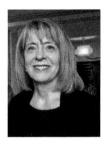

Margaret E. Wierman, MD
Editor

Over the last 10 years, there have been major advances in our understanding of the role of testosterone, DHEA, and other adrenal prohormones in the normal physiology of women as well as their role in pathologic disorders. Advances in accurate measurements of androgens have allowed revisiting of the definitions of "low, normal, and high" levels. This issue is focused on the latest research into what is "normal, high, and potentially low" and the implications of androgen excess or deficiency in various disorders. First, we review the physiology of androgens in women, define hyperandrogenism, and describe the differential diagnosis of disorders to consider in our patients in the clinic. Since polycystic ovarian syndrome (PCOS) is the most common cause of hyperandrogenism, the next articles examine the disorder across the lifespan. A review of the limitations of current definitions and criteria begins the issue. Then, an outline of the ontogeny of PCOS across puberty and adolescence with reference to animal models follows to attempt to further understand underlying mechanisms of disease. Since women with PCOS have a high risk of infertility, an article reviews updated guidelines on induction of ovulation in these women. An approach to preparing the PCOS patient for pregnancy and management across gestation is useful for clinicians. Then, we step back to review what is new in our understanding of the genetics of PCOS and whether these new advances alter our understanding of the variability of the clinical phenotype and risk features of individual patients. The complex interplay between metabolic and cardiovascular risk factors in women with PCOS is reviewed with an update on the latest international clinical guidelines on risk assessment and treatment. Last, in this section, the authors review the broader differential diagnosis in postmenopausal women who present with hyperandrogenism with a discussion of the spectrum of causes and treatment options. Next, a review of the major disorder of adrenal androgens in adults, nonclassical adrenal hyperplasia, is presented with up-to-date information on diagnosis, treatment, and new insights into the role of

Endocrinol Metab Clin N Am 50 (2021) xv–xvi
https://doi.org/10.1016/j.ecl.2020.12.004
0889-8529/21/© 2020 Published by Elsevier Inc.

multiple adrenal androgen precursors in clinical medicine. The last 2 articles then switch the focus to the current state of knowledge on the use of testosterone therapy for postmenopausal women with a current lack of data supporting its widespread administration and focused use in women with sexual dysfunction. Finally, we end with a review of the science of normal sexual function in women and discussion of whether androgens really play a role. Together, these topics, written by experts in the field, provide the student, fellow, clinician, and researcher insights into the role of androgens in women.

Margaret E. Wierman, MD
Division of Endocrinology, Diabetes
and Metabolism
Integrative Physiology
Pituitary Adrenal and
Neuroendocrine Tumor Program
University of Colorado Anschutz Medical Campus
Rocky Mountain Regional VAMC
Endocrinology MS8106
12801 East 17th Avenue, RC1S
Aurora, CO 80045, USA

E-mail address:
Margaret.wierman@CUAnschutz.edu

Hyperandrogenic Anovulation
Differential Diagnosis and Evaluation

Margaret E. Wierman, MD

KEYWORDS

- PCOS • CAH • Congenital adrenal hyperplasia • Androgen secreting tumors
- Cushing's syndrome

KEY POINTS

- Hyperandrogenic anovulation refers to the spectrum of disorders that present with clinical and/or biochemical signs and symptoms of excess androgens as well as irregular menses.
- A careful history of the timing of the onset, constellation of the symptoms and signs is critical to the appropriate diagnosis.
- Selected laboratory and/or radiologic testing allows a clinician to narrow the differential diagnostic categories.

INTRODUCTION

Women who present with irregular menses can be subdivided into those with or without accompanying features of acne and hirsutism, suggesting hyperandrogenic anovulation. The differential diagnosis, clinical presentation, and laboratory and radiologic evaluation of women with hyperandrogenic anovulation are outlined elsewhere in this article. A careful history as to the timing of the onset of the symptom complex, its pace and severity, physical examination for the pattern of acne and excessive hair growth, and signs of virilization or signs of other endocrine disorders is always needed. Together with the appropriate laboratory and radiologic evaluations, a clinician may make the appropriate diagnosis and chose the appropriate treatment options, depending on the patient's age, reproductive status, and goals.

CLINICAL PRESENTATION OF PATIENTS WITH HYPERANDROGENIC ANOVULATION

Most patients with hyperandrogenic anovulation seek medical care for signs of acne, abnormal hair growth, and irregular menses.

Diabetes and Metabolism Division, Department of Medicine, University of Colorado Anschutz Medical Campus, Rocky Mountain Regional Veterans Affairs Medical Center, University of Colorado School of Medicine, Endocrinology MS8106, 12801 East 17 Avenue, RC1S, Aurora, CO 80045, USA
E-mail address: Margaret.wierman@cuanschutz.edu

Endocrinol Metab Clin N Am 50 (2021) 1–10
https://doi.org/10.1016/j.ecl.2020.12.003
0889-8529/21/Published by Elsevier Inc.

endo.theclinics.com

Acne vulgaris is a disorder of the piloebaceous unit that includes comedones, inflammatory papules, and pustules with various degrees of scaring.[1] It usually presents in the prepubertal or peripubertal period with an incidence of up to 85%.[2] The prevalence decreases across adulthood with about 59% of women aged 20 to 29 compared with 26% of women aged 40 to 49.[3] Scarring from acne and the associated side effects are often accompanied by a poor self-image.[1] Acne is an androgen-dependent process in most women as demonstrated by the onset of acne in the pubertal period associated with increasing dehydroepiandrosterone sulfate (DHEAS) levels, and in adulthood with elevated total or free testosterone levels. In addition, acne usually responds to therapies that suppress androgens, such as oral contraceptives and androgen receptor antagonists. The proposed mechanism is that androgens activate the production of sebum production through androgen receptors on sebaceous glands.[1,2] All women with persistent acne should be evaluated for hyperandrogenism. Alternative causes of acneiform eruptions include allergic reaction to glucocorticoids, cosmetics, hair products, chemicals, and environmental exposures.[1,3]

Hirsutism is another frequent complaint from women presenting for evaluation of hyperandrogenic anovulation. About 70% of women with acne also have concomitant abnormal hair growth and more than 80% is androgen dependent.[4] Hirsutism is defined as abnormal terminal hair growth in a male pattern, in women.[5] This entity is to be distinguished from hypertrichosis, which is a more diffuse, generalized hair growth owing to genetic predisposition, or medications such as phenytoin or cyclosporine. In addition, diffuse villous hair may occur with anorexia and/or severe weight loss.

Different ethnicities, as outlined elsewhere in this article, have variability in terminal hair amounts and distribution, but hirsutism is defined in 9 specific areas, including the lip, chin, neck, upper chest, and upper lower abdomen (arms, legs, upper back, and buttocks). The degree of hair growth is often defined using the Ferriman–Gallwey score of more than the 95th percentile for that ethnic population[6] Caucasian and Black populations usually have a score of less than 8; Mediterranean, Hispanic, and Middle Eastern women of less than 10; South American of less than 6; and Asian women variably from less than 2 to less than 7.[4] There are limitations of the Ferriman–Gallwey score, including subjective scoring variability and a lack of consideration of excessive localized hair growth, yet no other scoring systems have been developed. Importantly, however, women notice even modest changes in hair growth and, if associated with irregular menses, the patients often have hyperandrogenism.[7] In summary, the mechanism of hirsutism is androgen action at the hair follicle to transition to terminal hairs in sex-specific regions. Because of the cyclic nature of hair growth in various regions, any intervention to alter facial hair takes more than 4 to 6 months, with a maximal effect of often more than 9 months.[4] Idiopathic hirsutism, in contrast, is defined as hirsutism in the absence of elevated androgens or irregular menses and is thought to be due to an increased sensitivity of the hair follicle to normal androgen levels.

Irregular menses is the third component of picture of women presenting with hyperandrogenic anovulation. There are many causes of irregular menses, either owing to a mechanical issue (ie, a cervical polyp or uterine fibroid) or more often, a hormonal disorder. Disturbances of the hypothalamic–pituitary–ovarian axis causing irregular or absent menses are common.

During the pubertal process, maturation of the reproductive axis in the female occurs such that the average age of menarche is 12 years or younger in most developed countries.[4,8] Precocious puberty is defined as menses earlier than age 8 years and delayed puberty is defined with onset of menarche after age 14 year. After the first menses, the intermenstrual interval is often shorter or longer than 28 days for about 12 to 18 months. Many disorders of the female reproductive axis may occur across pubertal development. On one extreme, absence of gonadotropin-releasing hormone–induced luteinizing hormone secretion may be observed owing to genetic forms of idiopathic hypogonadotropic hypogonadism or be acquired, as in young women with anorexia nervosa. More commonly, in up to 6% of women, less severe defects occur in patients with acquired hypothalamic amenorrhea.[4,8] The spectrum of these disorders present at one extreme with a failure to undergo puberty, or as secondary amenorrhea associated with eating disorders, excessive exercise, and low body weight after significant weight loss, as well as with stress.

Hypothalamic amenorrhea represents a group of disorders that present quite differently compared with the focus of this discussion, which is hyperandrogenic anovulation. Whereas women with hypothalamic amenorrhea usually have absent or short intermenstrual lengths, women with hyperandrogenic anovulation usually have irregular cycles with long intermenstrual periods. The spectrum of disorders included under hyperandrogenic anovulation are outlined in **Box 1**. The presenting features of each are discussed elsewhere in this article, and most of these disorders are discussed, in depth, in other articles.

DISORDERS THAT PRESENT WITH HYPERANDROGENIC ANOVULATION

Polycystic ovarian syndrome (PCOS) is the most common underlying disorder in women presenting with hyperandrogenic anovulation, occurring in 6% to 12% of women of reproductive age.[9–11] In a series of more than 1200 women evaluated for androgen excess in the United Kingdom, 89% of premenopausal and 29% of postmenopausal women were found to have PCOS.[12] Several international based definitions for PCOS have been described with the National Institutes of Health, Rotterdam, and Androgen Excess Society guidelines being the most commonly used. The National Institutes of Health definition includes clinical and/or biochemical evidence of hyperandrogenism, anovulation, and the exclusion of other disorders.[9,10] The Rotterdam criteria require only 2 of the following: clinical or biochemical hyperandrogenism, anovulation, and ovarian morphology on ultrasound examination, most recently defined as more than 20 follicles per ovary. The newest guideline by the Androgen Excess Society adds back the requirement for irregular menses to the Rotterdam definition to exclude women with hypothalamic amenorrhea who have cysts on their ovaries.[9–11] It is important to remember that in adolescence normal pubertal development includes a multifollicular ovarian morphology.[13]

To confirm a diagnosis of PCOS other disorders must be excluded, including nonclassical congenital adrenal hyperplasia, androgen-secreting tumors, hyperprolactinemia, Cushing's syndrome, obesity-related hyperandrogenism, and exogenous use of androgens.[10] A small subset of women with PCOS develop a more severe presentation of hyperandrogenism termed hyperthecosis, which is difficult to diagnose and must be differentiated from an ovarian or adrenal tumor.[5] The diagnosis and treatment of women with PCOS is critical because of the associated-long term complications of infertility, abnormal weight gain, metabolic syndrome, gestational diabetes, obstructive sleep apnea, hepatic steatosis, depression, stroke, and potential cardiovascular risk.[14,15]

Nonclassical congenital adrenal hyperplasia refers to the adult onset of hyperandrogenism in women with mutations in the genes encoding for enzyme in adrenal steroid hormone synthesis pathway, mostly commonly 21-hydroxylase.[16–18] Mutations in the CYP21A2 gene cause a block to cortisol production and excess sex hormone,

> **Box 1**
> **Differential diagnosis of hyperandrogenic anovulation**
>
> - Polycystic ovarian syndrome
> - Nonclassical congenital adrenal hyperplasia
> - Obesity-induced hyperandrogenic anovulation
> - Cushing's syndrome
> - Prolactinoma
> - Ovarian or adrenal tumor
> - Exogenous use of prohormones or androgens

predominantly androgen precursors, presenting as pubertal androgen excess. Whereas the incidence of classical congenital adrenal hyperplasia is 1:10 to 20,000, nonclassical congenital adrenal hyperplasia occurs in 0.1% to 0.2% of the Caucasian population and up to 1% to 4% of certain ethnic groups, such as Eastern European Jews or Middle Eastern populations. The diagnosis can be confirmed with evidence of an elevation in the 17-hydroxy progesterone levels in the follicular phase of a menstrual cycle (>200 ng/dL) or in response to adrenocorticotropic hormone stimulation (>1000 ng/dL).[16–18] Making the diagnosis of nonclassical congenital adrenal hyperplasia is important for optimal therapy for future fertility, as well as other long-term health outcomes.[19]

Obesity-induced hyperandrogenic anovulation is poorly defined and studied, but a clinically observed disorder in which women with a history of a normal menarche and regular menses, without acne or abnormal hair growth in adolescence, have either rapid or progressive weight gain, such as may occur with successive pregnancies. These patients often notice they hit a critical threshold weight (the converse of what is observed in the lower weight threshold noted by women with low body mass and weight loss) where they develop irregular menses or amenorrhea. However, in addition, a subset of these women then develop hirsutism and/or acne. The hypothesis is that the excess fat tissue produces both excess androgen precursors and estrogens. This finding is in contrast with some women who, with excessive weight gain, develop a hypothalamic amenorrhea picture, without signs of hyperandrogenism. Studies suggest that women with obesity-induced hyperandrogenic anovulation may have had a variant of PCOS before the weight gain that triggered the other manifestations.[20] Clinically, however, many of these women have a reversal of the phenotype if they are able to lose weight, which is uncommon in women with true PCOS.

Cushing's syndrome should always be excluded in women with hyperandrogenic anovulation. Excess cortisol from an exogenous source, or endogenous production from a pituitary adenoma producing adrenocorticotropic hormone, ectopic adrenocorticotropic hormone–producing tumors, or dysregulated adrenal production of cortisol must be considered.[21,22] Additional signs and symptoms are often present, including facial plethora, moon facies, supraclavicular fat pads, spontaneous ecchymoses, wide violaceous striae, changes in body weight distribution, sleep disturbance, proximal muscle weakness, and mood disorders.[21,22]

A prolactinoma is the most common type of pituitary tumor representing 40% of tumors and in up to 10% of amenorrheic women.[23,24] The tumors present with irregular menses or amenorrhea in women and more commonly with a hypothalamic amenorrhea pattern. However, some women with prolactinomas have associated hirsutism thought to be commonly associated with elevations in DHEAS levels. An elevated prolactin also may be caused by pregnancy, hypothyroidism or many different medications, such as antidepressants, antipsychotics, which must be considered.[23,24]

Ovarian or adrenal tumors that produce androgens are rare causes of hyperandrogenic anovulation.[25,26] These tumors usually present clinically with a more rapid onset and more severe signs and symptoms of hyperandrogenism. The hirsutism is usually more dramatic in its rate of growth and distribution in a male pattern, with associated anabolic appearance owing to testosterone or DHEAS levels in the male range. Other associated signs include male pattern baldness, breast atrophy, clitoromegaly, and voice deepening. Associated issues with worsening hypertension, hyperlipidemia and metabolic complications also may occur. Only 10% of ovarian tumors present with excess sex steroid hormone production.[25,26] These tumors usually secrete testosterone and sometimes androstenedione and estrogens. Differentiation from ovarian hyperthecosis is difficult if a transvaginal ultrasound examination does not demonstrate a discrete ovarian mass.[25,26] Adrenal tumors secrete cortisol or DHEAS, but rarely can produce testosterone; high levels would usually be in association with adrenal cortical carcinomas.[25]

Exogenous abuse of androgens must be considered in today's society where women are being prescribed or take off-label pharmacologic amounts of testosterone, dehydroepiandrosterone, or other prohormones. In addition, dehydroepiandrosterone and androstenedione are often contaminating substances in protein powders and supplements that are promoted by health food advocates. Because these supplements are not regulated by the US Food and Drug Administration or other governmental agencies, the amounts of the components or consistencies across batches are not known. Dehydroepiandrosterone and androstenedione themselves are not androgens, that is, they do not bind the androgen receptor, but can be converted into testosterone and in some cases to estradiol with adverse effects.[27,28] Competitive female athletes have been given or taken pharmacologic amounts of testosterone to improve performance with adverse effects. More recently, postmenopausal women have been given off-label testosterone formulations approved only for hypogonadal males, including testosterone gels, depo formations of injectable testosterone, or testosterone pellets to stimulate libido. Clinically, we are seeing women with testosterone levels in, or above, the normal male range, often with associated side effects, including hypertension, abnormal lipid profiles, male pattern balding, voice changes, and severe hirsutism (Wierman ME and Santoro N, unpublished observations, 2020). As a result, the Endocrine Society and the Institute of Medicine have recently recommended against this dangerous practice (Institute of Medicine webinar July 2020).

LABORATORY EVALUATION

The laboratory evaluation of a patient presenting with hyperandrogenic anovulation should include the tests outlined in **Box 2**. Testosterone is the major androgen produced by the ovary and best correlates with hyperandrogenism causing acne and hirsutism.[4,29,30] Testosterone is also secreted in smaller amounts by the adrenal glands and by peripheral tissues, including the liver and adipose tissue. In some cases, a free testosterone measured by dialysis is a more sensitive indicator of hyperandrogenism in women. Unfortunately, direct free testosterone levels available in most commercial assays are completely unreliable. Alternatively, free testosterone levels may be calculated using a total testosterone level and sex hormone–binding globulin level as outlined in the Endocrine Society's guideline on hirsutism.[4]

DHEAS is the other androgen to be measured. DHEAS is the major androgen prohormone produced by the adrenal glands.[29,30] Whereas the precursor dehydroepiandrosterone is pulsatile, short-lived, and increases with stress, DHEAS has a long half-life and reflects f adrenal androgen action. It is often slightly or moderately elevated in women with PCOS or adrenocorticotropic hormone–dependent Cushing's syndrome and extremely elevated in women with adrenocortical cancer (ie, >800 pg/mL); conversely, it is suppressed in women with adrenal Cushing's syndrome.

To diagnose nonclassical congenital adrenal hyperplasia, 17-hydroxyprogesterone should be measured in the follicular phase of the menstrual cycle or measured 30 minutes after administration of cosyntropin (250 μg) intravenously (if the basal level is borderline elevated).[17] Androstenedione is another adrenal prohormone that is elevated in patients with nonclassical congenital adrenal hyperplasia. It is not part of the diagnostic criteria, but can be a useful hormone to measure to monitor the efficacy of therapy.[17]

Measurement of the gonadotropins, luteinizing hormone, and follicle-stimulating hormone, drawn within the first 5 days after the onset of menses, or after the induction of menses with a progesterone withdrawal (medroxyprogesterone 5 mg for 7 days) is useful. Normal women or women with hypothalamic amenorrhea have low or low normal luteinizing hormone and follicle-stimulating hormone ratios in the early follicular phase, whereas many women with PCOS have high luteinizing hormone/follicle-stimulating hormone ratios (ie, >2.5) owing to a rapid gonadotropin-releasing hormone–induced luteinizing hormone secretory pattern.[20,31] In contrast, women with diminished ovarian reserve would have a high follicle-stimulating hormone/luteinizing hormone pattern.

Prolactin is measured to exclude disorders of elevated prolactin that can cause irregular menses.[23]

Hypercortisolism, causing Cushing's syndrome, can be evaluated with 3 potential screening tests. A dexamethasone suppression test can be performed in a woman not on exogenous estrogen therapy (because of the otherwise high false-positive test rate from estrogen-induced cortisol binding globulin and higher baseline cortisol levels). This dexamethasone suppression test entails taking a 1-mg tablet of dexamethasone between 11 PM and midnight the night before a 8 AM blood draw for cortisol.[21] A cortisol level of 1.8 mg/dL or lower excludes Cushing's syndrome. Alternatively, multiple salivary cortisol measurements, obtained at 11 PM, can be used as a screening test, as long as the patient does not have a sleep disorder causing physiologic hypercortisolism. Last, a 24-hour collection for urine free cortisol and creatinine measurement can used as a screening test, assuming normal kidney function. After establishing biochemical hypercortisolism, the morning adrenocorticotropic hormone and DHEAS levels determine if the etiology of Cushing's syndrome is an adrenocorticotropic hormone–dependent or independent process (ie, adrenocorticotropic hormone and DHEAS levels are generally high normal or frankly elevated in Cushing's disease owing to a pituitary or ectopic adrenocorticotropic hormone source, but both low normal or frankly low in a cortisol-secreting adrenal tumor).

RADIOLOGIC EVALUATION

Vaginal ultrasound examination is a standard component of confirming the diagnosis of PCOS, but is not required. Ovarian size of greater than 10 mL bilaterally or multiple follicles of more than 20 confirm PCOS morphology ovaries.[9] The transvaginal or transabdominal ultrasound examination is also useful in detecting the androgen

---

Box 2
Laboratory and radiologic testing in hyperandrogenic anovulation

Laboratory evaluation
- Testosterone: all patients
- DHEAS: all patients
- Androstenedione: to follow in patients with nonclassical congenital adrenal hyperplasia
- Luteinizing hormone and follicle-stimulating hormone timed in the first 5 days after onset of menses: useful to distinguish PCOS from hypothalamic amenorrhea or diminished ovarian reserve
- Prolactin: all patients
- Twenty-four–hour urinary cortisol, dexamethasone suppression test, and/or salivary cortisol: to exclude hypercortisolism
- Adrenocorticotropic hormone, cortisol, and DHEAS: useful in distinguishing adrenocorticotropic hormone-dependent or adrenocorticotropic hormone-independent Cushing's syndrome
- 17-Hydroxyprogesterone: random in follicular phase of the menstrual cycle or stimulated level in response to cosyntropin to diagnose nonclassical congenital adrenal hyperplasia

Radiologic evaluation
- Vaginal/pelvic ultrasound examination: component of the Rotterdam criteria for PCOS, or to detect an ovarian tumor
- MRI of the pituitary glands: to exclude a pituitary tumor
- Computed tomography scan of the abdomen: to exclude an adrenal tumor
- Other computed tomography scan of the chest, PET scans (FGD- or, 68 Ga-Dotatate) for ectopic tumors

---

producing ovarian tumors, which are often small. An MRI of the pelvis can be useful if the ultrasound examination results are equivocal.

An MRI of the pituitary, with and without contrast, is performed to exclude or diagnose a pituitary tumor. A computed tomography scan of the abdomen, with an adrenal protocol, is used to diagnose an adrenal adenoma or carcinoma. Rarely, conventional computed tomography scans of the chest or pelvis, or newer PET/single photon emission computed tomography imaging, such as with 68-Ga-dotatate, may help to identify ectopic hormone producing tumors. Surgical resection of any localized tumor, causing Cushing's syndrome, is then the preferred treatment of choice.

Ovarian vein sampling was used historically; however, the procedure is quite technically challenging and studies did not support its specificity in identifying the location of an ovarian tumor versus bilateral ovarian androgen production from hyperthecosis.[32]

SUMMARY

There is clinical usefulness in dividing patients who present with irregular menses or amenorrhea into those who have associated clinical and or biochemical signs of hyperandrogenism, including acne and hirsutism. This distinction allows the provider to obtain the appropriate history, perform a careful examination, and order the selected laboratory and radiologic tests to confirm the correct diagnosis and proceed to the appropriate therapeutic intervention. Other articles in this issue outline, in greater detail, the genetics and ontogeny of PCOS and the approach to fertility and care across pregnancy as well as the long-term complications including diabetes, obesity, and cardiovascular risk. Other topics include a discussion of nonclassical congenital adrenal hyperplasia and postmenopausal hyperandrogenism. In addition, the role of androgens in sexual function, the use of testosterone in postmenopausal women and the risks of testosterone therapy to women are reviewed.

CLINICS CARE POINTS

- Disorders of the female reproductive axis are common.
- When irregular menses is combined with clinical signs of hyperandrogenism the differential diagnosis can be narrowed to 7 disorders.
- Careful, history of the timing and pace of signs and symptoms are critical to the correct diagnosis.
- Laboratory tests usually performed include testosterone, DHEAS, prolactin, 17OH Progesterone with other tests chosen based on the differential diagnosis.

DISCLOSURE

None.

REFERENCES

1. Tan AU, Schlosser BJ, Paller AS. A review of diagnosis and treatment of acne in adult female patients. Int J Womens Dermatol 2018;4(2):56–71.
2. Bhate K, Williams HC. Epidemiology of acne vulgaris. Br J Dermatol 2013;168(3): 474–85.
3. Collier CN, Harper JC, Cafardi JA, et al. The prevalence of acne in adults 20 years and older. J Am Acad Dermatol 2008;58(1):56–9.
4. Martin KA, Anderson RR, Chang RJ, et al. Evaluation and treatment of hirsutism in premenopausal women: an Endocrine Society Clinical Practice Guideline. J Clin Endocrinol Metab 2018;103(4):1233–57.
5. Rosenfield RL. Clinical practice. Hirsutism. N Engl J Med 2005;353(24):2578–88.
6. Ferriman D, Gallwey JD. Clinical assessment of body hair growth in women. J Clin Endocrinol Metab 1961;21:1440–7.
7. Souter I, Sanchez LA, Perez M, et al. The prevalence of androgen excess among patients with minimal unwanted hair growth. Am J Obstet Gynecol 2004;191(6): 1914–20.
8. Rothman MS, Wierman ME. Female hypogonadism: evaluation of the hypothalamic-pituitary-ovarian axis. Pituitary 2008;11(2):163–9.
9. Azziz R, Carmina E, Dewailly D, et al. The Androgen Excess and PCOS Society criteria for the polycystic ovary syndrome: the complete task force report. Fertil Steril 2009;91(2):456–88.
10. Legro RS, Arslanian SA, Ehrmann DA, et al. Diagnosis and treatment of polycystic ovary syndrome: an Endocrine Society clinical practice guideline. J Clin Endocrinol Metab 2013;98(12):4565–92.
11. Walters KA, Gilchrist RB, Ledger WL, et al. New perspectives on the pathogenesis of PCOS: neuroendocrine origins. Trends Endocrinol Metab 2018;29(12): 841–52.
12. Elhassan YS, Idkowiak J, Smith K, et al. Causes, Patterns, and Severity of Androgen Excess in 1205 Consecutively Recruited Women. J Clin Endocrinol Metab 2018;103(3):1214–23.

13. Witchel SF, Burghard AC, Tao RH, et al. The diagnosis and treatment of PCOS in adolescents: an update. Curr Opin Pediatr 2019;31(4):562–9.
14. Kumarendran B, O'Reilly MW, Manolopoulos KN, et al. Polycystic ovary syndrome, androgen excess, and the risk of nonalcoholic fatty liver disease in women: a longitudinal study based on a United Kingdom primary care database. PloS Med 2018;15(3):e1002542.
15. Sanchez-Garrido MA, Tena-Sempere M. Metabolic dysfunction in polycystic ovary syndrome: pathogenic role of androgen excess and potential therapeutic strategies. Mol Metab 2020;35:100937.
16. Krone N, Dhir V, Ivison HE, et al. Congenital adrenal hyperplasia and P450 oxidoreductase deficiency. Clin Endocrinol (Oxf) 2007;66(2):162–72.
17. Speiser PW, Azziz R, Baskin LS, et al. Congenital adrenal hyperplasia due to steroid 21-hydroxylase deficiency: an Endocrine Society clinical practice guideline. J Clin Endocrinol Metab 2010;95(9):4133–60.
18. White PC, Speiser PW. Congenital adrenal hyperplasia due to 21-hydroxylase deficiency. Endocr Rev 2000;21(3):245–91.
19. Arlt W, Krone N. Adult consequences of congenital adrenal hyperplasia. Horm Res 2007;68(Suppl 5):158–64.
20. Welt CK, Carmina E. Clinical review: lifecycle of polycystic ovary syndrome (PCOS): from in utero to menopause. J Clin Endocrinol Metab 2013;98(12): 4629–38.
21. Lacroix A, Feelders RA, Stratakis CA, et al. Cushing's's syndrome. Lancet 2015; 386(9996):913–27.
22. Nieman LK, Biller BM, Findling JW, et al. Treatment of Cushing's's syndrome: an endocrine society clinical practice guideline. J Clin Endocrinol Metab 2015; 100(8):2807–31.
23. Melmed S, Casanueva FF, Hoffman AR, et al. Diagnosis and treatment of hyperprolactinemia: an Endocrine Society clinical practice guideline. J Clin Endocrinol Metab 2011;96(2):273–88.
24. Molitch ME, Drummond J, Korbonits M. Prolactinoma Management. [Updated 2018 Sep 30]. In: Feingold KR, Anawalt B, Boyce A, et al, editors. Endotext [Internet]. South Dartmouth (MA): MDText.com, Inc.; 2000. Available at: https://www.ncbi.nlm.nih.gov/books/NBK279174/.
25. Rothman MS, Wierman ME. How should postmenopausal androgen excess be evaluated? Clin Endocrinol (Oxf) 2011;75(2):160–4.
26. Shu S, Deng S, Tian JQ, et al. The clinical features and reproductive prognosis of ovarian neoplasms with hyperandrogenemia: a retrospective analysis of 33 cases. Gynecol Endocrinol 2019;35(9):825–8.
27. Borjesson A, Lehtihet M, Andersson A, et al. Studies of athlete biological passport biomarkers and clinical parameters in male and female users of anabolic androgenic steroids and other doping agents. Drug Test Anal 2020;12(4): 514–23.
28. Havnes IA, Jorstad ML, McVeigh J, et al. The anabolic androgenic steroid treatment gap: a national study of substance use disorder treatment. Subst Abuse 2020;14. 1178221820904150.
29. Wierman ME, Arlt W, Basson R, et al. Androgen therapy in women: a reappraisal: an Endocrine Society clinical practice guideline. J Clin Endocrinol Metab 2014; 99(10):3489–510.

30. Wierman ME, Basson R, Davis SR, et al. Androgen therapy in women: an Endocrine Society Clinical Practice guideline. J Clin Endocrinol Metab 2006;91(10): 3697–710.
31. Martin K, Santoro N, Hall J, et al. Clinical review 15: management of ovulatory disorders with pulsatile gonadotropin-releasing hormone. J Clin Endocrinol Metab 1990;71(5). 1081A–1081G.
32. Hickman LC, Goodman L, Falcone T. Value of selective venous catheterization in the diagnosis of hyperandrogenism. Fertil Steril 2017;108(6):1085.

Diagnosis of Polycystic Ovary Syndrome
Which Criteria to Use and When?

Sydney Chang, MD[a], Andrea Dunaif, MD[b],*

KEYWORDS

- Polycystic ovary syndrome • PCOS • Hyperandrogenism • Diagnostic criteria
- Disease classification

KEY POINTS

- Current diagnostic criteria for polycystic ovary syndrome (PCOS) are based on expert opinion, the lowest level of evidence. There has never been a formal consensus process to determine criteria for the diagnosis of PCOS.
- Individual diagnostic criteria have limitations that may result in misclassification of National Institutes of Health (NIH) and non-NIH Rotterdam PCOS phenotypes.
- Although current criteria have identified 2 major groups (NIH and non-NIH Rotterdam) that have different metabolic risks, recent genetic analyses have suggested that these criteria do not identify biologically distinct PCOS subtypes.
- Diagnosis of PCOS, therefore, should depend on management goals. The assessment of polycystic ovarian morphology is not needed to manage the endocrine and metabolic features of PCOS but is critical for reproductive endocrinologists managing infertility associated with PCOS.
- Agnostic data mining approaches have identified PCOS subtypes (metabolic and reproductive) that appear genetically distinct, potentially providing a biologically meaningful way to establish criteria for the diagnosis of PCOS.

WHAT IS POLYCYSTIC OVARY SYNDROME ?

PCOS is a highly heritable complex genetic disorder.[1] It is the most common disorder of reproductive-aged women, affecting up to 15% of this population worldwide, depending on the diagnostic criteria applied.[2,3] PCOS is a leading cause of anovulatory infertility, obesity, and type 2 diabetes mellitus.[3,4] It is a syndrome, a collection of signs and features, of unknown etiology. Despite its high prevalence and major

[a] Department of Obstetrics and Gynecology, Division of Reproductive Endocrinology, Zucker School of Medicine at Hofstra/Northwell, 210A E 64th St. 1st Floor, New York, NY 10065, USA;
[b] Department of Medicine, Division of Endocrinology, Diabetes and Bone Disease, Icahn School of Medicine at Mount Sinai, Atran Building, 1428 Madison Avenue, 4th Floor, Room 4-36, New York, NY 10029, USA
* Corresponding author. One Gustave L. Levy Place, Box 1055, New York, NY 10029.
E-mail address: andrea.dunaif@mssm.edu

Endocrinol Metab Clin N Am 50 (2021) 11–23
https://doi.org/10.1016/j.ecl.2020.10.002
0889-8529/21/© 2020 Elsevier Inc. All rights reserved.

morbidities, affected women remain remarkably underserved.[1] Diagnosis frequently is delayed[5] and physicians often are poorly informed about PCOS.[6]

PCOS is characterized by enhanced luteinizing hormone (LH) relative to follicle-stimulating hormone release, increased LH-dependent ovarian testosterone (T) production, frequent adrenal androgen excess, profound insulin resistance, dysglycemia, and obesity.[1,3] Antimüllerian hormone levels are increased in PCOS, and recent rodent[7] and human[8] studies suggest antimüllerian hormone plays a direct role in PCOS pathogenesis.

Polycystic ovarian morphology (PCOM) is characterized by an excessive number of antral follicles, which may be the result of accelerated follicle growth and/or prolonged survival of small follicles.[9,10] Additional hallmarks of PCOM are ovarian stromal hypertrophy, theca cell hyperplasia, and ovarian cortical thickening.[11] Theca cells in women with polycystic ovaries secrete more androgens, basally and in response to LH and insulin.[12] Abnormalities of both theca and granulosa cells may contribute to the arrest of follicular development seen in PCOS.[12–14]

DIAGNOSTIC CRITERIA
National Institutes of Health Criteria

Stein and Leventhal[15] generally are credited with the original description in 1935 of what has come to be known as PCOS, although there are clear reports of the disorder dating back to Hippocrates in the fifth century BCE.[16] It was not until 1990, however, that there was a formal effort to develop standard diagnostic criteria as part of a meeting of experts in medical and reproductive endocrinology sponsored by the NIH.[17] The participants were asked to vote on the potential diagnostic features of PCOS; features receiving the most votes, clinical and/or biochemical evidence of hyperandrogenism (HA) and ovulatory dysfunction (OD) with the exclusion of secondary causes, became known as the NIH criteria.[17] These criteria did not include PCOM because, even at that time, it was recognized that PCOM was present in 20% to 30% of women with regular menses and no hyperandrogenic symptoms.[18] The prevalence of PCOS has been constant, at 5% to 8%, using the NIH criteria.[19]

Rotterdam Criteria

In 2003, the European Society of Human Reproduction and Embryology and the American Society for Reproductive Medicine (ASRM) sponsored another meeting of experts in Rotterdam, Netherlands, during which PCOM was added as a diagnostic criterion.[20,21] The Rotterdam criteria required 2 of the 3 features for the diagnosis of PCOS: (1) OD, (2) HA, and (3) PCOM. The intent of the Rotterdam criteria was to encompass the NIH criteria as well as to broaden the definition of PCOS. The result was 2 new phenotypes, HA + PCOM and OD + PCOM (**Fig. 1**). The prevalence of PCOS using the Rotterdam criteria is as high as approximately 15% of reproductive-aged women.[22,23]

Androgen Excess Society Criteria

In 2006, the Androgen Excess Society (now known as the Androgen Excess and PCOS Society [AE-PCOS]) convened another task force of experts.[24] This group recommended that HA should be a requirement for the diagnosis of PCOS, which limited the diagnosis of PCOS to 3 of the 4 Rotterdam phenotypes: HA + OD + PCOM, HA + OD, and HA + PCOM.[24,25] The AE-PCOS criteria have never been widely adopted.

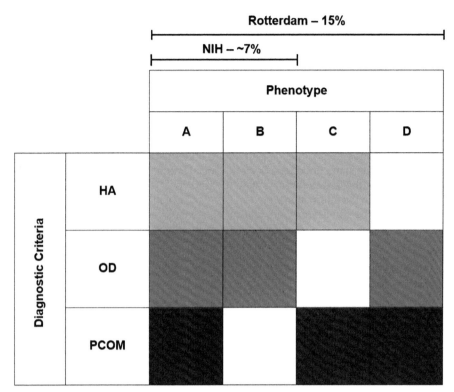

Fig. 1. Comparing components of different diagnostic criteria. NIH PCOS must include both HA + OD, ± PCOM. There are no endocrine or metabolic differences between phenotypes A and B; there is no need to assess PCOM in NIH PCOS. Rotterdam criteria require at least 2 of the 3 criteria to be present, adding 2 new phenotypes HA + PCOM and OD + PCOM. The prevalence of PCOS increases from approximately 7% to 15% when including the 2 non-NIH Rotterdam phenotypes.

National Institutes of Health–Sponsored Evidence-Based Methodology Workshop on Polycystic Ovary Syndrome

In 2012, the NIH sponsored an evidence-based methodology workshop on PCOS to review the current state of the science in the field.[26] This meeting differed from the previous PCOS meetings in that it followed a formal consensus process. Although it was not an official NIH Consensus Development Conference (https://consensus.nih.gov/), the meeting followed the same court model, where the evidence is presented to a panel that functions as a jury. The panel consisted of individuals who are experts in their fields (gynecology, diabetes and metabolism, cardiology, and primary care) but are not engaged in PCOS research, allowing independent assessment of the scientific evidence by an unbiased panel. The panel's final report noted that "the name 'PCOS' was a distraction and an impediment to progress," and that the emphasis on PCOM created confusion because it was neither necessary nor sufficient for the diagnosis of PCOS.[26] They recommended using the Rotterdam criteria with precise specification of phenotype (see **Fig. 1**) and proposed a comprehensive research agenda that included assessment of the epidemiology and long-term health outcomes of the PCOS phenotypes.

Evidence-Based Guidelines

Consensus conferences since have been replaced by evidence-based guidelines for the diagnosis and management of PCOS, such as those published in 2013 by the Endocrine Society[27] and the 2018 international evidence-based guidelines.[28–30] The quality of the evidence on which these guidelines are based, however, is predominantly low due to a paucity of randomized clinical trials (RCTs). Unfortunately, the key research initiatives recommended by the 2012 Evidence-based Methodology Workshop on Polycystic Ovary Syndrome to critically assess the utility of the PCOS diagnostic criteria as well as the optimal therapies and long-term health outcomes have not been undertaken, in large part due to underfunding of the field.[31] Of the 34 recommendations in the Endocrine Society Clinical Practice Guideline,[27] the evidence supporting 24 of these was rated as "low" or "very low." There were almost 175 recommendations in the international guideline,[28–30] of which only 31 were ranked as evidence based; the remainder were clinical consensus recommendations or clinical practice points.

LIMITATIONS OF THE INDIVIDUAL DIAGNOSTIC CRITERIA
Hyperandrogenism

Clinical hyperandrogenism
Signs of HA in women include hirsutism, acne, and alopecia. Male pattern terminal hair growth is a fairly reliable indicator of androgen action.[32] The development of hirsutism is determined by number of pilosebaceous units and their sensitivity to androgen action, which genetically are determined and vary by race and ethnicity.[32,33] Although increased male pattern terminal hair growth assessed by ethnicity-specific Ferriman-Gallwey scores is pathognomonic for HA, as many as 50% of HA women do not have clinically significant terminal hair growth.[34] Furthermore, women often remove unwanted hair using mechanical methods. Acne and alopecia can reflect HA but are not reliable enough to use as surrogate markers for androgen excess.[35,36]

Biochemical hyperandrogenism
Hyperandrogenemia is characterized by elevated circulating endogenous androgen levels. T circulates specifically bound to sex hormone–binding globulin (SHBG) and loosely associated with albumin; only approximately 1% of circulating T is free T (FT).[37] Both FT and albumin-associated T are biologically available[37] and are referred to collectively as non-SHBG bound T (NSB-T). FT is elevated in approximately 70% of women with PCOS.[25] NSB-T, however, provides a better index of T that is bioavailable.[38]

The main limitation of biochemical HA as a diagnostic criterion is that it can be difficult to detect at the lower circulating levels present in women and children.[39] Measuring T is challenging because steroids structurally are similar, and antibodies used in immunoassays can cross-react with other steroids.[39] The gold standard for measuring total T (TT) is liquid chromatography followed by tandem mass spectrometry (LC/MS-MS)[39]; this is the method recommended by the Endocrine Society[39] and the Centers for Disease Control and Prevention.[40] Unfortunately, some clinical laboratories still use inaccurate TT assays, such as electrochemiluminescence immunoassays, performed directly on serum or plasma (direct assays).[39] These methods lack sensitivity and specificity and should not be used,[39] especially in women and children.

The gold standard for measuring FT is equilibrium dialysis; however, it is expensive, cumbersome, and subject to variability if not correctly performed.[39] Direct FT assays are unreliable and should not be used.[39] Therefore, guidelines[25,39] recommend calculating FT and NSB-T based on the binding affinity of T to SHBG and albumin utilizing the law of mass action.[41] It is possible to order calculated FT and NSB-T as part of T profiles offered by clinical laboratories. It also is easy to perform these calculations using measured TT and SHBG values (e.g. http://www.issam.ch/freetesto.htm); albumin levels can be assumed to be normal.[41] The accuracy of these calculations depend on the quality of the TT assay.[39] Unreliable TT assays may lead to a failure to detect biochemical HA and result in misclassification of NIH PCOS as the non-NIH Rotterdam OD + PCOM phenotype (**Table 1**).

Assessment of HA should include measurement of dehydroepiandrosterone sulfate (DHEAS) because a substantial minority of women with HA have isolated DHEAS elevations.[25] DHEAS also is a marker of adrenal androgen-secreting neoplasms. Measurement of androstenedione does not increase the detection of HA in most cases.[42] Recently, 11-oxygenated C19 steroids, such as 11β-hydroxyandrostenedione, have been recognized as an important pool of circulating adrenal androgens,[43] including in women with PCOS.[44] Nevertheless, there is no current evidence to suggest that these steroids should be included in the clinical assessment of HA.[45]

Ovulatory Dysfunction

Among women with PCOS who report regular menstrual cycles, 20% to 30% have been found to have anovulatory cycles with biochemical assessment of ovulation.[24,25] Oligomenorrhea (defined as <6–8 menstrual cycles per year) is virtually pathognomonic for anovulation, but more frequent cycles do not necessarily indicate ovulation. A recent study of greater than 600,000 menstrual cycles revealed that there is more variation within normal menstrual cycles than previously recognized,[46] suggesting that it may be difficult to determine ovulatory status based solely on self-report of 21-day to 35-day cycles. To increase detection of anovulatory cycles, the ASRM recommends that women with other signs of PCOS who report regular menstrual cycles undergo ovulatory monitoring using basal body temperatures or measurement of a serum progesterone level in the luteal phase.[47] Lack of confirmation of ovulation can lead to misclassification of NIH PCOS as the ovulatory non-NIH Rotterdam HA + PCOM phenotype (see **Table 1**).

Polycystic Ovarian Morphology

Despite the intrinsic abnormalities seen in PCO,[9–11] the presence of PCOM is neither necessary nor sufficient for diagnosis of PCOS.[18,48] There is no evidence that the presence of PCOM has any implications with regard to the endocrine or metabolic features of PCOS.[27,49] There also is no evidence to support the addition of assessment of PCOM to the diagnosis of NIH PCOS. The international evidence-based guidelines state that ultrasound is not needed for the diagnosis of PCOS in women with HA + OD.[28–30] Similarly, the Endocrine Society guideline for the management of hirsutism states that demonstrating PCOM to diagnose ovulatory PCOS (HA + PCOM) is unlikely to affect management of hirsutism.[50] Furthermore, PCOM is so common in adolescents that ultrasound is not recommended for the diagnosis of PCOS in this age range.[28–30,42,51]

Ovarian ultrasound is a critical component of assisted reproductive technology (ART), because assessment of antral follicle count predicts ovarian responses to medications[52] as well as risk of ovarian hyperstimulation syndrome.[53] All women undergoing infertility evaluation and treatment routinely have pelvic ultrasounds at baseline and throughout their treatment to monitor follicular growth. The detection of PCOM is dependent on the sensitivity of the ultrasound equipment, the skill of the operator, the approach (vaginal vs abdominal), and the weight of the patient.[28–30] Furthermore,

Table 1
Misclassification of Rotterdam polycystic ovarian syndrome phenotypes

	Hyperandrogenism	Ovulatory Dysfunction	Polycystic Ovarian Morphology	Interpretation
Each criteria appropriately assessed	√	√	√	NIH phenotype
HA not detected due to use of incorrect TT or FT assay	X	√	√	Non-NIH Rotterdam phenotype
Anovulation not detected due to reported regular menses	√	X	√	Non-NIH Rotterdam phenotype
Ovarian morphology not detected due to technology, operator, or patient factors	√	√	X	NIH phenotype

ovarian ultrasound examinations performed by clinical radiologists frequently do not use the Rotterdam criteria to interpret their findings. Therefore, it is challenging for medical endocrinologists to obtain an accurate ovarian ultrasound assessment of PCOM. In summary, assessment of PCOM is not needed for the endocrine management of PCOS or hirsutism; access to accurate ovarian sonography is limited outside of reproductive endocrinology.

Polycystic Ovary Syndrome Phenotypes

Application of the Rotterdam criteria results in 4 PCOS phenotypes: (A) HA + OD + PCOM, (B) HA + OD, (C3) HA + PCOM, and (D) OD + PCOM (see **Fig. 1**). Phenotypes A and B also are known as NIH PCOS; phenotypes C and D also are known as non-NIH Rotterdam PCOS. There is no evidence, however, that there are endocrine or metabolic differences between HA + OD and HA + OD + PCOM.[27,49] Thus, there is no rationale for stratifying HA + OD cases by the presence of absence of PCOM. Stratification by the presence or absence of hirsutism has been proposed in the Androgen Excess Society guidelines,[24] adding 12 potential phenotypes. Hirsutism is a distinct biologic process related to androgen action and there are insufficient data to support using it to further subgroup PCOS.[50]

TOWARD A BIOLOGICAL BASIS FOR POLYCYSTIC OVARY SYNDROME CLASSIFICATION

Current Polycystic Ovary Syndrome Classification

Michael Crichton stated, "the work of science has nothing whatever to do with consensus. Consensus is the business of politics. Science, on the contrary, requires only one investigator who happens to be right...consensus is evoked only in situations where the science is not solid enough."[54] Despite labeled as consensus criteria, all the PCOS diagnostic criteria are based on expert opinion—the lowest level of evidence.[55] As better scientific evidence accumulates, consensus no longer is necessary. Unfortunately, the newer so-called evidence-based PCOS guidelines[27–30] still are largely based on expert opinion because of the paucity of high-quality RCTs addressing most features of PCOS.[31]

Validation of Diagnostic Criteria

Diagnostic criteria should identify discrete biologically meaningful subgroups that are stratified by associated disease risk, biomarker profiles, responses to treatment, and/or genetic architecture. The consistent difference among the PCOS phenotypes is the severity of insulin resistance. It has been well established that the NIH PCOS phenotype is at higher risk for insulin resistance and associated metabolic abnormalities compared with non-NIH Rotterdam PCOS phenotypes.[3,56,57] Ovulatory PCOS (HA + PCOM) tend to have lower body mass index (BMI) than the NIH phenotype[58] and have either mild or no metabolic abnormalities.[59]

Although current criteria have identified 2 major subgroups (NIH vs non-NIH Rotterdam) with differing metabolic risk, a recent well-powered meta-analysis of PCOS genome-wide association studies (GWAS) has suggested that current criteria do not identify genetically distinct subgroups.[60] GWAS permit the agnostic interrogation of the entire genome for regions that are associated with a given trait or disease and provide insight into causal pathways.[61] GWAS in PCOS case-control cohorts of Han Chinese and European ancestry have implicated pathways regulating gonadotropin secretion and action, androgen biosynthesis, insulin resistance, and ovarian aging in the pathogenesis of PCOS.[1,62,63] The largest genetic analysis of PCOS to date—a GWAS meta-analysis that contained greater than 10,000 PCOS cases and 100,000 controls—compared NIH, non-NIH Rotterdam, and self-reported PCOS and found no significant differences in genetic architecture for 13 of 14 identified loci.[60] There was 1 locus that was associated significantly more strongly with NIH PCOS than with non-NIH Rotterdam and self-reported PCOS,[60] which suggests that this locus is involved in pathways regulating insulin action because NIH PCOS are more insulin resistant than the other PCOS phenotypes. This meta-analysis suggests that, overall, the genetic architecture of NIH PCOS, non-NIH Rotterdam PCOS and self-reported PCOS is similar.

Objective Approaches to Polycystic Ovary Syndrome Classification

Cluster analysis is a well-established mathematical approach to aggregate traits into clusters of similar data. Cluster analysis increasingly is applied to large biomedical datasets to identify subtypes of disorders, such as type 2 diabetes mellitus.[64] The authors performed unsupervised hierarchical cluster analysis in women of European ancestry with PCOS diagnosed by NIH criteria using quantitative anthropometric, reproductive, and metabolic traits and identified 2 distinct clusters, designated *reproductive* and *metabolic* (**Fig. 2**).[65] The reproductive subtype had higher LH and SHBG levels with relatively low BMI and insulin levels, whereas the metabolic subtype had higher BMI, glucose, and insulin levels with lower SHBG and LH levels.[65] The authors replicated these clusters in an independent cohort of European ancestry NIH PCOS cases. GWAS was performed limiting the cases to the reproductive or metabolic subtypes. Five novel susceptibility loci were discovered, 4 associated with the reproductive subtype and 1 associated with the metabolic subtype.[65] The authors' findings suggest that these subtypes are biologically relevant because they appear to have distinct genetic architectures. This study presents an objective, unbiased mathematical approach to PCOS classification and validates this approach by demonstrating that the reproductive and metabolic subtypes thus identified are associated with novel and distinct gene regions. These PCOS subtypes need to be replicated in PCOS diagnosed by Rotterdam criteria as well as in PCOS cohorts of non-European ancestry.

Which Polycystic Ovary Syndrome Diagnostic Criteria to Use When

The NIH criteria of HA + OD are sufficient to detect women at high risk of insulin resistance and associated metabolic abnormalities.[3] The presence of PCOM has no impact on the diagnosis or endocrine management of NIH PCOS. In contrast, ovulatory women with HA are at low risk for insulin resistance and associated metabolic abnormalities, whether or not they have PCOM.[3,56] Therefore, medical endocrinologists should focus on determining whether an HA patient is ovulatory. Usually, OD is not a subtle finding as it is accompanied by oligomenorrhea (<6–8 menses per year). Because a substantial minority of women reporting regular menstrual cycles may be anovulatory, however, it is prudent to confirm ovulation in this subgroup of HA patients.[47] Glucose tolerance and lipid levels should be evaluated in NIH PCOS.[3,27,66]

Symptom-based management for hirsutism, or for acne and alopecia with biochemically documented HA, can be undertaken in ovulatory women without additional metabolic screening.[3] As highlighted in the Endocrine Society guideline for the management of hirsutism, establishing a diagnosis of Rotterdam PCOS by assessing ovarian morphology does not affect management.[50] There is no evidence, however, to support the use of the Rotterdam criteria for the diagnosis of PCOS, that is, the addition of PCOM, for the management of endocrine or metabolic features of PCOS. In contrast, treatment of anovulatory infertility associated with PCOS using ART requires monitoring of ovarian morphology. Assessment of HA is important for establishing a diagnosis of NIH PCOS because these patients require monitoring for

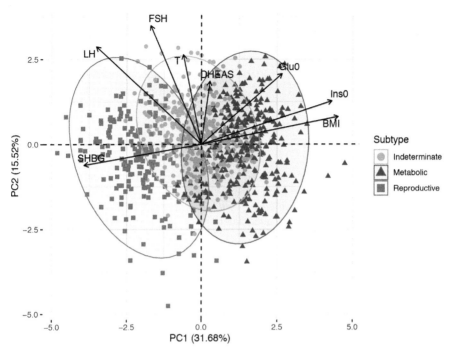

Fig. 2. Principal component analysis plot of quantitative traits for a genotyped PCOS clustering cohort showing a biologically driven method of PCOS classification. Women with PCOS were clustered into distinct groups—metabolic, reproductive, and indeterminate—based on BMI, fasting insulin, fasting glucose, DHEAS, T, follicle-stimulating hormone, LH, SHBG, and genotype data. The relative magnitude and direction of trait correlations with the principal components are shown with black arrows. Glu0, fasting glucose; Ins0, fasting insulin; PC, principal component. (*From* Dapas M, Lin FTJ, Nadkarni GN, et al. Distinct subtypes of polycystic ovary syndrome with novel genetic associations: An unsupervised, phenotypic clustering analysis. PLoS Med. 2020;17(6):e1003132; with permission.)

associated metabolic abnormalities. The presence or absence of HA, however, does not affect short-term reproductive management.

SUMMARY

The diagnostic criteria for PCOS are based on expert opinion and do not identify genetically distinct subgroups of women. Furthermore, each individual diagnostic criterion has limitations that may lead to misclassification between PCOS phenotypes. The endocrine management of PCOS does not require assessment of ovarian morphology. Unsupervised cluster analysis of clinical and biochemical traits has shown promise in identifying genetically distinct metabolic and reproductive PCOS subtypes. Such objective approaches enable the transition from PCOS classification based on expert opinion, which is subjective, to classification based on demonstrable biologic differences.

CLINICS CARE POINTS

- Hirsutism is sufficient to diagnose HA but not all HA women are hirsute.
- Acne and alopecia are not reliable markers of HA.

- LC/MS-MS assay is needed for accurate TT measurement. FT and NSB-T should be calculated based on TT and SHBG.
- Women presenting with HA who report regular menses should undergo testing to confirm ovulation.
- Ovarian morphology is not needed for the endocrine management of PCOS.

DISCLOSURE

The authors have nothing to disclose.

REFERENCES

1. Dunaif A. Perspectives in Polycystic Ovary Syndrome: From Hair to Eternity. J Clin Endocrinol Metab 2016;101(3):759–68.
2. Carmina E, Lobo RA. Polycystic ovary syndrome (PCOS): arguably the most common endocrinopathy is associated with significant morbidity in women. J Clin Endocrinol Metab 1999;84(6):1897–9.
3. Diamanti-Kandarakis E, Dunaif A. Insulin resistance and the polycystic ovary syndrome revisited: an update on mechanisms and implications. Endocr Rev 2012; 33(6):981–1030.
4. Rubin KH, Glintborg D, Nybo M, et al. Development and Risk Factors of Type 2 Diabetes in a Nationwide Population of Women With Polycystic Ovary Syndrome. J Clin Endocrinol Metab 2017;102(10):3848–57.
5. Gibson-Helm M, Teede H, Dunaif A, et al. Delayed Diagnosis and a Lack of Information Associated With Dissatisfaction in Women With Polycystic Ovary Syndrome. J Clin Endocrinol Metab 2017;102(2):604–12.
6. Lin AW, Bergomi EJ, Dollahite JS, et al. Trust in Physicians and Medical Experience Beliefs Differ Between Women With and Without Polycystic Ovary Syndrome. J Endocr Soc 2018;2(9):1001–9.
7. Tata B, Mimouni NEH, Barbotin AL, et al. Elevated prenatal anti-Müllerian hormone reprograms the fetus and induces polycystic ovary syndrome in adulthood. Nat Med 2018;24(6):834–46.
8. Gorsic LK, Kosova G, Werstein B, et al. Pathogenic Anti-Müllerian Hormone Variants in Polycystic Ovary Syndrome. J Clin Endocrinol Metab 2017;102(8):2862–72.
9. Webber LJ, Stubbs S, Stark J, et al. Formation and early development of follicles in the polycystic ovary. Lancet 2003;362(9389):1017–21.
10. Webber LJ, Stubbs SA, Stark J, et al. Prolonged survival in culture of preantral follicles from polycystic ovaries. J Clin Endocrinol Metab 2007;92(5):1975–8.
11. Hughesdon PE. Morphology and morphogenesis of the Stein-Leventhal ovary and of so-called "hyperthecosis". Obstet Gynecol Surv 1982;37(2):59–77.
12. Gilling-Smith C, Willis DS, Beard RW, et al. Hypersecretion of androstenedione by isolated thecal cells from polycystic ovaries. J Clin Endocrinol Metab 1994;79(4): 1158–65.
13. Mason HD, Willis DS, Beard RW, et al. Estradiol production by granulosa cells of normal and polycystic ovaries: relationship to menstrual cycle history and concentrations of gonadotropins and sex steroids in follicular fluid. J Clin Endocrinol Metab 1994;79(5):1355–60.
14. Willis DS, Watson H, Mason HD, et al. Premature response to luteinizing hormone of granulosa cells from anovulatory women with polycystic ovary syndrome: relevance to mechanism of anovulation. J Clin Endocrinol Metab 1998;83(11):3984–91.
15. Stein IF, Leventhal ML. Amenorrhea associated with bilateral polycystic ovaries. Am J Obstet Gynecol 1935;29:181–91.

16. Azziz R, Dumesic DA, Goodarzi MO. Polycystic ovary syndrome: an ancient disorder? Fertil Steril 2011;95(5):1544–8.
17. Zawadzki JK, Dunaif A. Diagnostic criteria for polycystic ovary syndrome: towards a rational approach. In: Dunaif A, Givens JR, Haseltine FP, et al, editors. Polycystic ovary syndrome. Boston (MA): Blackwell Scientific Inc; 1992. p. 377–84.
18. Polson DW, Adams J, Wadsworth J, et al. Polycystic ovaries–a common finding in normal women. Lancet 1988;1(8590):870–2.
19. Bozdag G, Mumusoglu S, Zengin D, et al. The prevalence and phenotypic features of polycystic ovary syndrome: a systematic review and meta-analysis. Hum Reprod 2016;31(12):2841–55.
20. Rotterdam ESHRE/ASRM-Sponsored PCOS consensus workshop group. Revised 2003 consensus on diagnostic criteria and long-term health risks related to polycystic ovary syndrome (PCOS). Hum Reprod 2004;19(1):41–7.
21. Rotterdam ESHRE/ASRM-Sponsored PCOS consensus workshop group. Revised 2003 consensus on diagnostic criteria and long-term health risks related to polycystic ovary syndrome. Fertil Steril 2004;81(1):19–25.
22. Fauser BC, Tarlatzis BC, Rebar RW, et al. Consensus on women's health aspects of polycystic ovary syndrome (PCOS): the Amsterdam ESHRE/ASRM-Sponsored 3rd PCOS Consensus Workshop Group. Fertil Steril 2012;97(1):28–38.e5.
23. March WA, Moore VM, Willson KJ, et al. The prevalence of polycystic ovary syndrome in a community sample assessed under contrasting diagnostic criteria. Hum Reprod 2010;25(2):544–51.
24. Azziz R, Carmina E, Dewailly D, et al. Positions statement: criteria for defining polycystic ovary syndrome as a predominantly hyperandrogenic syndrome: an Androgen Excess Society guideline. J Clin Endocrinol Metab 2006;91(11):4237–45.
25. Azziz R, Carmina E, Dewailly D, et al. The Androgen Excess and PCOS Society criteria for the polycystic ovary syndrome: the complete task force report. Fertil Steril 2009;91(2):456–88.
26. NIH. Evidence-based Methodology Workshop on Polycystic Ovary Syndrome. presented at: 2012-EXECUTIVE SUMMARY (Final Report). 2012. Available at: https://prevention-archive.od.nih.gov/docs/programs/pcos/FinalReport.pdf. Accessed March 10, 2020.
27. Legro RS, Arslanian SA, Ehrmann DA, et al. Diagnosis and treatment of polycystic ovary syndrome: an Endocrine Society clinical practice guideline. J Clin Endocrinol Metab 2013;98(12):4565–92.
28. Teede HJ, Misso ML, Costello MF, et al. Recommendations from the international evidence-based guideline for the assessment and management of polycystic ovary syndrome. Fertil Steril 2018;110(3):364–79.
29. Teede HJ, Misso ML, Costello MF, et al. Recommendations from the international evidence-based guideline for the assessment and management of polycystic ovary syndrome. Clin Endocrinol (Oxf) 2018;89(3):251–68.
30. Teede HJ, Misso ML, Costello MF, et al. Recommendations from the international evidence-based guideline for the assessment and management of polycystic ovary syndrome. Hum Reprod 2018;33(9):1602–18.
31. Brakta S, Lizneva D, Mykhalchenko K, et al. Perspectives on Polycystic Ovary Syndrome: Is Polycystic Ovary Syndrome Research Underfunded? J Clin Endocrinol Metab 2017;102(12):4421–7.
32. Paparodis R, Dunaif A. The Hirsute woman: challenges in evaluation and management. Endocr Pract 2011;17(5):807–18.

33. Lee HJ, Ha SJ, Lee JH, et al. Hair counts from scalp biopsy specimens in Asians. J Am Acad Dermatol 2002;46(2):218–21.

34. Azziz R, Ehrmann D, Legro RS, et al. Troglitazone improves ovulation and hirsutism in the polycystic ovary syndrome: a multicenter, double blind, placebo-controlled trial. J Clin Endocrinol Metab 2001;86(4):1626–32.

35. Moradi Tuchayi S, Makrantonaki E, Ganceviciene R, et al. Acne vulgaris. Nat Rev Dis Primers 2015;1:15029.

36. Lin RL, Garibyan L, Kimball AB, et al. Systemic causes of hair loss. Ann Med 2016;48(6):393–402.

37. Rosenfield R, Moll G. The role of proteins in the distribution of plasma androgens and estradiol. In: Molinatti G, Martini L, James V, editors. Androgenization in women. New York: Raven Press; 1983. p. 25–45.

38. Manni A, Pardridge WM, Cefalu W, et al. Bioavailability of albumin-bound testosterone. J Clin Endocrinol Metab 1985;61(4):705–10.

39. Rosner W, Auchus RJ, Azziz R, et al. Position statement: Utility, limitations, and pitfalls in measuring testosterone: an Endocrine Society position statement. J Clin Endocrinol Metab 2007;92(2):405–13.

40. CDC. CDC Hormone Standardization Program (CDC HoSt). Available at: https://www.cdc.gov/labstandards/pdf/hs/CDC_Certified_Testosterone_Assays-508.pdf. Accessed July 29, 2020.

41. Vermeulen A, Verdonck L, Kaufman JM. A critical evaluation of simple methods for the estimation of free testosterone in serum. J Clin Endocrinol Metab 1999; 84(10):3666–72.

42. Goodman NF, Cobin RH, Futterweit W, et al. American Association of Clinical Endocrinologists, American College of Endocrinology, and androgen excess and PCOS society disease state clinical review: guide to the best practices in the evaluation and treatment of polycystic ovary syndrome–part 1. Endocr Pract 2015;21(11):1291–300.

43. Rege J, Nakamura Y, Satoh F, et al. Liquid chromatography-tandem mass spectrometry analysis of human adrenal vein 19-carbon steroids before and after ACTH stimulation. J Clin Endocrinol Metab 2013;98(3):1182–8.

44. O'Reilly MW, Kempegowda P, Jenkinson C, et al. 11-Oxygenated C19 Steroids Are the Predominant Androgens in Polycystic Ovary Syndrome. J Clin Endocrinol Metab 2017;102(3):840–8.

45. Pretorius E, Arlt W, Storbeck KH. A new dawn for androgens: Novel lessons from 11-oxygenated C19 steroids. Mol Cell Endocrinol 2017;441:76–85.

46. Bull JR, Rowland SP, Scherwitzl EB, et al. Real-world menstrual cycle characteristics of more than 600,000 menstrual cycles. NPJ Digit Med 2019;2:83.

47. Practice Committee of the American Society for Reproductive Medicine. The evaluation and treatment of androgen excess. Fertil Steril 2006;86(5 Suppl 1):S241–7.

48. Murphy MK, Hall JE, Adams JM, et al. Polycystic ovarian morphology in normal women does not predict the development of polycystic ovary syndrome. J Clin Endocrinol Metab 2006;91(10):3878–84.

49. Johnstone EB, Rosen MP, Neril R, et al. The polycystic ovary post-rotterdam: a common, age-dependent finding in ovulatory women without metabolic significance. J Clin Endocrinol Metab 2010;95(11):4965–72.

50. Martin KA, Anderson RR, Chang RJ, et al. Evaluation and Treatment of Hirsutism in Premenopausal Women: An Endocrine Society Clinical Practice Guideline. J Clin Endocrinol Metab 2018;103(4):1233–57.

51. Screening and Management of the Hyperandrogenic Adolescent: ACOG Committee Opinion, Number 789. Obstet Gynecol 2019;134(4):e106–14.

52. Ng EH, Tang OS, Ho PC. The significance of the number of antral follicles prior to stimulation in predicting ovarian responses in an IVF programme. Hum Reprod 2000;15(9):1937–42.

53. Steward RG, Lan L, Shah AA, et al. Oocyte number as a predictor for ovarian hyperstimulation syndrome and live birth: an analysis of 256,381 in vitro fertilization cycles. Fertil Steril 2014;101(4):967–73.

54. Crichton M. Aliens Cause Global Warming. The Caltech Michelin Lecture, Jan 17, 2003. 2003. Available at: https://stephenschneider.stanford.edu/Publications/PDF_Papers/Crichton2003.pdf.

55. US Preventative Services Task Force. Guide to clinical preventive services: report of the U.S. Preventive services task force. Darby (PA): Diane Publishing; 1989.

56. Dunaif A, Graf M, Mandeli J, et al. Characterization of groups of hyperandrogenic women with acanthosis nigricans, impaired glucose tolerance, and/or hyperinsulinemia. J Clin Endocrinol Metab 1987;65(3):499–507.

57. Moghetti P, Tosi F, Bonin C, et al. Divergences in insulin resistance between the different phenotypes of the polycystic ovary syndrome. J Clin Endocrinol Metab 2013;98(4):E628–37.

58. Wild RA, Carmina E, Diamanti-Kandarakis E, et al. Assessment of cardiovascular risk and prevention of cardiovascular disease in women with the polycystic ovary syndrome: a consensus statement by the Androgen Excess and Polycystic Ovary Syndrome (AE-PCOS) Society. J Clin Endocrinol Metab 2010;95(5):2038–49.

59. Carmina E, Chu MC, Longo RA, et al. Phenotypic variation in hyperandrogenic women influences the findings of abnormal metabolic and cardiovascular risk parameters. J Clin Endocrinol Metab 2005;90(5):2545–9.

60. Day F, Karaderi T, Jones MR, et al. Large-scale genome-wide meta-analysis of polycystic ovary syndrome suggests shared genetic architecture for different diagnosis criteria. PLoS Genet 2018;14(12):e1007813.

61. Guo X, Rotter JI. Genome-Wide Association Studies. JAMA 2019;322(17):1705–6.

62. Day FR, Hinds DA, Tung JY, et al. Causal mechanisms and balancing selection inferred from genetic associations with polycystic ovary syndrome. Nat Commun 2015;6:8464.

63. Hayes MG, Urbanek M, Ehrmann DA, et al. Genome-wide association of polycystic ovary syndrome implicates alterations in gonadotropin secretion in European ancestry populations. Nat Commun 2015;6:7502.

64. Ahlqvist E, Storm P, Käräjämäki A, et al. Novel subgroups of adult-onset diabetes and their association with outcomes: a data-driven cluster analysis of six variables. Lancet Diabetes Endocrinol 2018;6(5):361–9.

65. Dapas M, Lin FTJ, Nadkarni GN, et al. Distinct subtypes of polycystic ovary syndrome with novel genetic associations: An unsupervised, phenotypic clustering analysis. PLoS Med 2020;17(6):e1003132.

66. Goodman NF, Cobin RH, Futterweit W, et al. American Association of Clinical Endocrinologists, American College of Endocrinology, and androgen excess and PCOS society disease state clinical review: guide to the best practices in the evaluation and treatment of polycystic ovary syndrome - part 2. Endocr Pract 2015;21(12):1415–26.

Polycystic Ovary Syndrome
Ontogeny in Adolescence

Christine M. Burt Solorzano, MD[a,b],
Christopher R. McCartney, MD[a,c],*

KEYWORDS

- PCOS • Puberty • Hyperandrogenism • Hyperandrogenemia • Daughters
- Premature pubarche • Premature adrenarche • Obesity

KEY POINTS

- The initial manifestations of PCOS often arise during or shortly after puberty, presumably related to the pubertal increase in gonadotropins and, in turn, ovarian androgen production.
- The pubertal ontogeny of PCOS is difficult to study in humans because the pathophysiology is typically well entrenched before the diagnosis can be substantiated.
- Several groups seem to be at higher risk for developing adolescent PCOS (daughters of women with PCOS, girls with premature pubarche, and girls with obesity) and the study of these groups can offer insight into the pubertal ontogeny of PCOS.
- Available data support the hypothesis that the pubertal development of PCOS involves various combinations of genetic predisposition, intrauterine programming, hyperinsulinism, and other abnormalities, that provoke reproductive symptoms (eg, hyperandrogenism, ovulatory dysfunction) in response to the pubertal increase in gonadotropin secretion.

INTRODUCTION: THE CHALLENGE OF STUDYING NASCENT POLYCYSTIC OVARY SYNDROME

Polycystic ovary syndrome (PCOS) is characterized by hyperandrogenism, ovulatory dysfunction, and polycystic ovarian morphology (PCOM); it is also associated with metabolic comorbidities, such as obesity and insulin resistance.[1] PCOS is a complex, multigenic disorder with important environmental determinants, but its causes remain poorly understood.[2–4]

[a] Center for Research in Reproduction, University of Virginia School of Medicine, OMS Suhling Building, Room 6921, Hospital Drive, Charlottesville, VA 22908, USA; [b] Department of Pediatrics, Division of Endocrinology and Metabolism, University of Virginia School of Medicine, University of Virginia Health, Box 800386, Charlottesville, VA 22908, USA; [c] Department of Medicine, Division of Endocrinology and Metabolism, University of Virginia School of Medicine, University of Virginia Health, Box 801406, Charlottesville, VA 22908, USA
* Corresponding author. Center for Research in Reproduction, University of Virginia School of Medicine, OMS Suhling Building, Room 6921, Hospital Drive, Charlottesville, VA 22908.
E-mail address: CM2HQ@hscmail.mcc.virginia.edu

Endocrinol Metab Clin N Am 50 (2021) 25–42
https://doi.org/10.1016/j.ecl.2020.10.003
0889-8529/21/© 2020 Elsevier Inc. All rights reserved.
endo.theclinics.com

The pathophysiology of symptomatic PCOS generally unfolds across puberty, the developmental stage during which increases in pulsatile gonadotropin-releasing hormone (GnRH) release and gonadotropin secretion drive ovarian sex steroid production and follicular development, with the eventual establishment of highly complex feedback relationships that govern cyclic ovulation. However, the pubertal ontogeny of PCOS has been difficult to study because PCOS cannot be diagnosed before puberty, and diagnostic criteria appropriate for pubertal girls remain elusive.[4,5] For example, pubertal hyperandrogenemia has not been clearly defined, hirsutism takes time to develop, oligomenorrhea in the 1 to 2 years after menarche is not by itself considered abnormal, and there are no validated criteria for PCOM in adolescent girls.

By the time a diagnosis of adolescent PCOS is substantiated, the pathophysiology of PCOS seems to be largely, if not fully, entrenched. However, several groups seem to be at higher risk for developing adolescent PCOS (daughters of women with PCOS [PCOS-d], girls with premature pubarche, and girls with obesity) and the study of such groups can offer important insights into the pubertal ontogeny of PCOS.

CAUSES OF POLYCYSTIC OVARY SYNDROME: A BRIEF OVERVIEW

Some of the most carefully studied aspects of PCOS pathophysiology relate to abnormal ovarian function, insulin resistance and hyperinsulinemia, neuroendocrine dysfunction, and genetics. Additional factors include epigenetic modifications, adipose tissue dysfunction, inflammation, increased sympathetic nerve activity, environmental exposures, the microbiome, and so forth.[2–4] The multitude of contributing factors likely play different relative roles in different subsets of patients with PCOS.

Abnormal Ovarian Steroidogenesis and Folliculogenesis

Adolescents and adults with PCOS exhibit abnormal patterns of sex steroid secretion (eg, exaggerated 17-hydroxyprogesterone and androstenedione secretion) in response to acute GnRH agonist or human chorionic gonadotropin administration.[3] Abnormal steroidogenesis seems to be a stable property of ovarian theca cells in PCOS, partly reflecting increased expression of a splice variant of the DENND1A gene.[3] Similar abnormalities of adrenal sex steroid secretion are observed after exogenous corticotropin administration, suggesting a more global dysregulation of steroidogenesis in PCOS.[3] Such abnormalities are exacerbated by such factors as hyperinsulinemia and disordered gonadotropin secretion.[2]

PCOS is also characterized by abnormal follicular dynamics (enhanced follicular recruitment and later follicular arrest), which partly accounts for PCOM and likely involves, among other factors, abnormal gonadotropin action, intraovarian androgen excess, and hyperinsulinemia.[2,3,6] Moreover, antimüllerian hormone (AMH) concentrations, derived from granulosa cells in preantral and small antral ovarian follicles (2–9 mm), are approximately two- to four-fold elevated in PCOS.[7]

Insulin Resistance and Hyperinsulinemia

Women and adolescents with PCOS demonstrate metabolic insulin resistance that is exacerbated by, but partly independent of, obesity.[8] Insulin resistance may be further exacerbated during puberty, in part related to activation of the growth hormone axis.[4] The resulting compensatory hyperinsulinemia augments ovarian and adrenal androgen production, reduces hepatic sex hormone-binding globulin (SHBG) production (increasing androgen bioavailability), and disrupts ovarian follicular dynamics and function.[8] Genetic studies implicate several metabolism-related genes including INSR (insulin receptor), INS-VNTR (insulin gene variable number of tandem repeats), and IRS1 (Insulin

Receptor Substrate-1)[9]; and a recent mendelian randomization study suggested that a genetic risk score for fasting insulin is associated with an increased risk of PCOS.[10]

Reproductive Neuroendocrine Dysfunction

PCOS is associated with relative luteinizing hormone (LH) excess and follicle-stimulating hormone (FSH) deficiency, both of which promote ovarian hyperandrogenism and impair follicular development.[11] Genetic studies support the relevance of genes related to gonadotropin secretion and action in PCOS, including *FSHB* (FSH subunit beta), *FSHR* (FSH receptor), and *LHCGR* (LH/choriogonadotropin receptor).[9] Abnormal gonadotropin secretion in part relates to persistently high GnRH pulse frequency which in part reflects relative GnRH pulse generator resistance to negative feedback.[11] Although such negative feedback defects are programmed by prenatal exposure to androgen excess, they seem to require ongoing androgen action in adulthood.[11] Recent studies also imply the potential role of AMH in the GnRH neuron dysfunction of PCOS.[12,13]

Insight from Animal Models with Polycystic Ovary Syndrome–Like Features

Investigators have developed several animal models with PCOS-like features,[6] which permit invasive assessments and experimental manipulation that would be impractical, ethically unacceptable, or both in girls and women. Although no animal model perfectly replicates PCOS, such animal models have substantially informed the understanding of PCOS pathophysiology.

Prenatally androgenized (PNA) female rhesus macaques, sheep, and rodents demonstrate many PCOS-like features as adults.[6] For example, adult PNA female monkeys exhibit endogenous hyperandrogenemia, ovulatory dysfunction, polyfollicular ovaries, rapid GnRH pulsatility resistant to sex steroid negative feedback, abnormal gonadotropin secretion, increased adiposity, insulin resistance, impaired β-cell function, and dyslipidemia.[6] Yet complete or partial androgen receptor knockout prevents PCOS-like manifestations in PNA mice,[14] suggesting the primacy of androgens in this regard. Recent findings in mice also suggest that the effects of prenatal androgenization are transmitted through the germline in a transgenerational manner.[15] Although it remains unclear whether prenatal androgenization plays a role in PCOS, some human studies have supported this notion.[6,11]

Other animal models have been instructive. For example, peripubertal dihydrotestosterone treatment in female rodents produces many PCOS-like features, such as ovulatory dysfunction, polyfollicular ovaries, increased adiposity, and insulin resistance.[6] Of interest, neuron-specific androgen receptor knockout prevented many of the untoward effects of postnatal dihydrotestosterone,[16] suggesting the importance of central nervous system involvement in the pathophysiology of PCOS.

STUDIES IN GIRLS AT RISK FOR DEVELOPING POLYCYSTIC OVARY SYNDROME

Within the ethical and practical limitations accompanying pediatric research, investigators have assessed the pubertal ontogeny of PCOS by characterizing the development of abnormalities in girls at high risk for adolescent PCOS: PCOS-d, girls with a history of premature pubarche, and girls with obesity.

Daughters of Women with Polycystic Ovary Syndrome

PCOS-d are expected to share PCOS susceptibility gene variants with their mothers, may be exposed to an intrauterine environment that enhances PCOS risk, and are likely to share postnatal environmental exposures with their mothers. A large Swedish registry study suggested that PCOS-d are approximately five times more likely to be diagnosed with PCOS as adults compared with control daughters; and a longitudinal cohort study suggested that Chilean PCOS-d are 10-fold more likely than control daughters to develop PCOS according to Rotterdam criteria.[15]

Chilean daughters born to women with PCOS phenotype A (ie, with hyperandrogenism, oligo-/amenorrhea, and PCOM) have been characterized in several studies (**Table 1**).[17–25] As infants, these PCOS-d exhibited high serum AMH concentrations and exaggerated LH and estradiol responses to acute GnRH agonist stimulation.[17,22] During childhood, Chilean PCOS-d exhibited elevated serum AMH, ovarian enlargement, and lower serum FSH concentrations.[17,19–21] Although Chilean PCOS-d had no demonstrable hyperandrogenemia during childhood, a study of 1- to 3-year-old US PCOS-d suggested increased 5α-reductase activity.[26] Moreover, Chilean PCOS-d exhibited exaggerated 17-hydroxyprogesterone and dehydroepiandrosterone (DHEA) responsiveness to exogenous corticotropin during childhood (ages 4–8 years) and the peripubertal years (9–13 years), and approximately a third had exaggerated adrenarche.[21] Both AMH and ovarian volume seemed to be elevated throughout puberty in Chilean PCOS-d.[20,24] However, many of the classic reproductive abnormalities of PCOS (elevated testosterone, free androgen index, basal LH, LH/FSH ratio; lower SHBG; and exaggerated 17-hydroxyprogesterone and testosterone responses to acute GnRH agonist challenge) manifested only toward the end of puberty (eg, Tanner stage 4).[20,24,25]

Studies in peripubertal PCOS-d from the United States have supported some, but not all of the previously mentioned findings (**Table 2**).[26–30] In two US studies of prepubertal and early pubertal PCOS-d, AMH levels were not significantly elevated compared with control subjects, whereas estimates of free testosterone were increased.[28,30] Another study suggested no differences in urinary steroids, urinary gonadotropins, or ovarian volume in peripubertal PCOS-d.[29]

PCOS-d also exhibit early metabolic abnormalities (see **Tables 1** and **2**). For example, Chilean PCOS-d exhibit exaggerated serum insulin responses to an oral glucose challenge during childhood and puberty, despite no clear anthropometric abnormalities (eg, body mass index [BMI] z score, waist-to-hip ratio).[17–21,23–25] Similarly, female 8- to 14-year-old peripubertal first-degree relatives of US women with PCOS exhibited insulin resistance, exaggerated insulin responses to an oral glucose load, and impaired β-cell function, differences that remained after adjusting for differences in BMI z score.[27]

Girls with Premature and/or Exaggerated Adrenarche

Adrenarche represents the developmental rise in adrenal androgen production, heralded clinically by the development of pubic hair (pubarche), axillary hair, and apocrine odor.[31] Premature pubarche, occurring earlier than age 8 years in girls, is typically related to premature/exaggerated adrenarche and is a common cause of androgen excess in prepubertal children.[31,32]

Premature and/or exaggerated adrenarche may also represent a harbinger of PCOS. Ibanez and colleagues[33] initially observed that approximately half of Catalan (northeastern Spanish) girls with premature pubarche developed postpubertal oligomenorrhea, hirsutism, hyperandrogenemia, and functional ovarian hyperandrogenism in response to acute GnRH agonist testing. The emergence of PCOS-like abnormalities across puberty was assessed in several subsequent studies (**Table 3**).[34–39] Prepubertal Catalan girls with a history of premature pubarche exhibited elevated free androgen index, DHEA sulfate, and insulin-like growth factor-1 (IGF-1); hyperinsulinemia after an oral glucose load; and increased total and central adiposity despite

Table 1
Selected findings in Chilean daughters of women with PCOS

Putative Feature of PCOS	Infancy (Age 2–3 mo) References[17,22]	Mid to Late Childhood; Prepubertal References[17,18,20,21,23,24]	Early Puberty (Tanner 2–3) References[20,23,24]	Late Puberty (Tanner 4–5 and/or Postmenarcheal) References[20,23–25]	Peripubertal (Age 8–16 y, Tanner 1–5) References[18,19,21]
Higher total testosterone	–	–	–	+	+
Lower sex hormone–binding globulin	–	–	–	+	+/–
Higher free testosterone estimate	–	–	–	+	+
Higher androstenedione	–	–	–	–	–
Higher 17-hydroxyprogesterone	–	–	–	(–)	–
Higher dehydroepiandrosterone sulfate	–	–	–		+
More hirsutism	–	–	–	+	
Exaggerated 17-hydroxyprogesterone responsiveness (GnRH agonist)	–	–	–	+/–	
Exaggerated androstenedione responsiveness (GnRH agonist)	+	–	–	+	
Exaggerated testosterone responsiveness (GnRH agonist)	–	–	–	+/–	
Exaggerated estradiol responsiveness (GnRH agonist)	+				
Exaggerated 17-hydroxyprogesterone responsiveness (exogenous corticotropin)		+			+
Exaggerated dehydroepiandrosterone responsiveness (exogenous corticotropin)		+			+
Higher LH	–	–	–	(–)	–
Lower FSH	–	(–)	–	–	–

(continued on next page)

Table 1
(continued)

Putative Feature of PCOS	Infancy (Age 2–3 mo) References[17,22]	Mid to Late Childhood; Prepubertal References[17,18,20,21,23,24]	Early Puberty (Tanner 2–3) References[20,23,24]	Late Puberty (Tanner 4–5 and/or Postmenarcheal) References[20,23-25]	Peripubertal (Age 8–16 y, Tanner 1–5) References[18,19,21]
Higher LH-to-FSH ratio		–	–	(–)	
Higher GnRH agonist-stimulated LH	+	–		+	
Higher antimüllerian hormone	+	+	+	+	+
Greater ovarian volume		+	+	+	+
Greater global adiposity (eg, BMI z score)	–	–	–	–	–
Higher waist circumference	–	–	–	–	–
Higher waist-to-hip ratio	–	–	–	–	–
Higher fasting insulin		–	–	(–)	–
Higher fasting glucose		–	–	–	–
Higher insulin after oral glucose load		+	+	+	+
Insulin resistance by oral glucose tolerance test		–	–	+/–	
Higher triglycerides		–	–	+/–	+
Lower adiponectin		+	–	–	–
Higher leptin		–	–	–	–

Abbreviations: +, available data suggest presence; +/–, data mixed; (–), most but not all data suggest against presence; –, available data suggest against presence; blank, data not reported in these studies; BMI, body mass index.
Data from Refs.[17-25]

Table 2

Selected findings in North American daughters (PCOS-d) or first-degree relatives (PCOS-fdr) of women with PCOS

Putative Feature of PCOS	Young Childhood (Age 1–3 y) PCOS-d from Illinois Reference[26]	Prepubertal and Early Pubertal (Age 8–12 y; Tanner 1–3; Premenarcheal) PCOS-d and PCOS-fdr from Illinois and Pennsylvania References[28,30]	Midchildhood (Prepubertal) PCOS-d from Pennsylvania Reference[29]	Early Pubertal (Tanner 2–3)	Late Pubertal (Tanner 4–5)	Peripubertal (Age 8–14 y) PCOS-fdr from Quebec, Canada Reference[27]
Higher total testosterone (serum or urine)	+/−	+/−	−	−	−	−
Lower sex hormone–binding globulin		+/−				+
Higher free testosterone estimate		+				
Higher androstenedione (serum or urine)		−	−	−	−	−
Higher 17-hydroxyprogesterone (serum or urine)			−	−	−	−
Higher dehydroepiandrosterone sulfate (serum or urine)		−	−	−	−	
Increased apparent 5α-reductase activity	+					
Increased apparent 11β-hydroxysteroid dehydrogenase activity	−					
Hirsutism					+	
Higher LH (serum or urine)			−	−	−	
Lower FSH (serum or urine)			−	−		
Higher LH-to-FSH ratio (urine)			−	−	−	
Higher antimüllerian hormone			−	−	−	
Greater ovarian volume			−	−	−	

(continued on next page)

Table 2
(continued)

Putative Feature of PCOS	Young Childhood (Age 1–3 y) PCOS-d from Illinois Reference[26]	Prepubertal and Early Pubertal (Age 8–12 y; Tanner 1–3; Premenarcheal) PCOS-d and PCOS-fdr from Illinois and Pennsylvania References[28,30]	Midchildhood (Prepubertal) PCOS-d from Pennsylvania Reference[29]	Early Pubertal (Tanner 2–3) PCOS-d from Pennsylvania Reference[29]	Late Pubertal (Tanner 4–5) PCOS-d from Pennsylvania Reference[29]	Peripubertal (Age 8–14 y) PCOS-fdr from Quebec, Canada Reference[27]
Greater global adiposity (eg, BMI z score)	+	+/−	−	−	−	+
Increased central adiposity		−		+/−	−	−
Higher fasting insulin		−				+
Higher fasting glucose		−				−
Higher insulin after oral glucose load (serum or saliva)		−		−		+
Insulin resistance by oral glucose tolerance test						+
Abnormal β-cell function by oral glucose tolerance test						+
Insulin resistance by frequently sampled intravenous glucose tolerance test		−				+
Abnormal β-cell function by frequently sampled intravenous glucose tolerance test	+					+
High triglycerides		−				−
Low adiponectin						−
High leptin						+

Abbreviations: +, available data suggest presence; +/−, data mixed; −, available data suggest against presence; blank, data not reported in these studies; BMI, body mass index; PCOS-fdr, first-degree relatives of women with PCOS.

Table 3
Selected findings in Catalan girls with a history of premature pubarche

Putative Feature of PCOS	Mid to Late Childhood; Prepubertal References[35-37,39]	Early Puberty (Tanner 2; Premenarcheal) References[34-37,39]	Early/Midpuberty (Tanner 3; Premenarcheal) References[34-37,39]	Late Puberty (Tanner 4-5 and Postmenarcheal) References[34-39]
Higher total testosterone	+	–	+/–	+
Lower sex hormone–binding globulin	+/–	+/–	+/–	+
Higher free testosterone estimate	+	–	+	+
Higher androstenedione		–	–	+
Higher 17-hydroxyprogesterone		–	–	+/–
Higher dehydroepiandrosterone sulfate	+	+	–	(+)
Higher peak 17-hydroxypregnenolone (GnRH agonist)		+	–	+
Exaggerated 17-hydroxypregnenolone responsiveness (GnRH agonist)		–	+	+
Higher peak dehydroepiandrosterone (GnRH agonist)		+	+	+/–
Exaggerated dehydroepiandrosterone responsiveness (GnRH agonist)		+	–	+/–
Higher peak 17-hydroxyprogesterone (GnRH agonist)		–	–	+/–
Exaggerated 17-hydroxyprogesterone responsiveness (GnRH agonist)		–	–	+/–
Higher peak androstenedione (GnRH agonist)		–	–	+
Exaggerated androstenedione responsiveness (GnRH agonist)		–	–	+/–
Higher peak testosterone (GnRH agonist)		–	–	+
Higher peak estradiol (GnRH agonist)		–	–	+

(continued on next page)

Table 3
(continued)

Putative Feature of PCOS	Mid to Late Childhood; Prepubertal References[35–37,39]	Early Puberty (Tanner 2; Premenarcheal) References[34–37,39]	Early/Midpuberty (Tanner 3; Premenarcheal) References[34–37,39]	Late Puberty (Tanner 4–5 and Postmenarcheal) References[34–39]
Exaggerated 17-hydroxyprogesterone responsiveness (exogenous corticotropin)				−
Exaggerated androstenedione responsiveness (exogenous corticotropin)				+
Exaggerated dehydroepiandrosterone responsiveness (exogenous corticotropin)				+
Higher LH		−	−	+/−
Lower FSH		−	−	−
Higher GnRH agonist-stimulated LH	−	−	(−)	−
Greater global adiposity (eg, BMI)	+	(−)	(−)	+
Higher waist-to-hip ratio	+	+	+	+
Total body fat mass (dual-energy x-ray absorptiometry)	+	+	+	+
Percentage fat mass (dual-energy x-ray absorptiometry)	+	+	+	+
Truncal fat mass (dual-energy x-ray absorptiometry)	+	+	−	+
Abdominal fat mass (dual-energy x-ray absorptiometry)	+	+	+	+
Higher fasting insulin	+	−	−	+
Higher insulin after oral glucose load	+	+	+	+
Insulin resistance by oral glucose tolerance test	−	−	+/−	+/−
Higher IGF-1	+	−	−	−
Lower IGFBP-1	+	−	−	+
Higher triglycerides	+/−	+/−	+/−	+

Abbreviations: + available data suggest presence; (+), most but not all data suggest presence; +/−, data mixed; (−), most but not all data suggest against pres-

normal BMI. These latter two abnormalities were observed throughout puberty. Although elevations in total testosterone, free androgen index, and androstenedione were not observed in early puberty, hyperandrogenemia was demonstrable in later puberty. Similarly, although such girls demonstrated variably elevated 17-hydroxypregnenolone and DHEA responses to acute GnRH agonist stimulation throughout puberty, the more typical findings of functional ovarian hyperandrogenism (eg, exaggerated 17-hydroxyprogesterone and androstenedione responses to acute GnRH agonism) were not apparent until late puberty.[34] Abnormal ovulatory dysfunction became evident after 3 years postmenarche.[40]

A quarter to a third of women with PCOS have evidence for adrenal hyperandrogenemia,[41] and the potent androgen 11-ketotestosterone predominates among circulating androgens in girls with premature adrenarche and in women with PCOS.[42,43] Accordingly, the link between premature/exaggerated adrenarche and PCOS may partly reflect general abnormalities of androgen steroidogenesis, manifesting as adrenal hyperandrogenemia at adrenarche and ovarian hyperandrogenemia at puberty. Premature/exaggerated adrenarche and adolescent PCOS are also linked to increased visceral fat, hyperinsulinemia, and increased free IGF-1 concentrations, with the latter two augmenting adrenal and ovarian theca cell androgen production.[3,39,44–48] In Catalan girls with premature pubarche, a history of small for gestational age (SGA) was associated with a more severe phenotype in late puberty.[37] In these girls, peripubertal treatment with metformin reduced total and visceral adiposity, IGF-1 levels, and reduced the risk of hyperandrogenism, oligomenorrhea, and PCOS.[49–51]

Peripubertal Girls with Obesity

Obesity is associated with menstrual dysfunction and higher free testosterone concentrations in women with and without PCOS, and weight loss can ameliorate the manifestations of PCOS in adolescents and adults with obesity.[52] Additionally, PCOS has been associated with a high prevalence of obesity,[53] although referral bias partly accounts for this finding.[54] In a large population-based study of 15- to 19-year-old adolescent girls in the United States, the prevalence of PCOS was estimated to be 3.0-, 6.7-, and 14.7-fold elevated in girls with overweight, moderate obesity, and more extreme obesity, respectively.[55] Furthermore, in a large meta-analysis of PCOS cases and control subjects of European descent, linkage disequilibrium-score regression suggested that childhood obesity and BMI are genetically correlated with an increased risk of PCOS.[10] Mendelian randomization analyses also suggest that genetic risk scores for BMI are associated with PCOS.[10,56,57]

Free testosterone levels are approximately two- to four-fold higher in peripubertal girls with obesity compared with nonobese control subjects.[30,58–62] One study suggested that total testosterone was four-fold elevated in prepubertal girls with obesity,[58] whereas another suggested that free testosterone was more than eight-fold elevated in prepubertal girls with obesity, with absolute levels similar to those in Tanner 5 girls without obesity.[59] Although some studies imply that higher free testosterone is largely attributable to reduced SHBG in these girls,[30,62] others also demonstrated elevated total testosterone,[58,59,61] suggesting increased production. Some[58,61,63] but not all[30,62] studies suggest that peripubertal obesity is also associated with adrenal hyperandrogenemia.

Obesity presumably contributes to the pubertal ontogeny of PCOS partly via insulin resistance and compensatory hyperinsulinemia.[62] Some investigators have hypothesized that either SGA (intrauterine growth retardation) with postnatal catch-up growth and/or excessive postnatal weight gain in non-SGA children contributes to hepatovisceral fat excess, which increases risk for premature pubarche and PCOS via insulin resistance, hyperinsulinemia, IGF-1 excess, and hypoadiponectinemia.[64,65] Moreover, excess adiposity may be associated with altered peripheral steroid metabolism that can enhance hyperandrogenemia (eg, increased 17β-hydroxysteroid dehydrogenase type 5 activity, increased 5α-reductase activity, altered cortisol metabolism).[52]

Available data suggest that early pubertal girls with obesity exhibit reduced LH release without the expected overnight changes in LH pulse frequency and amplitude,[66–69] whereas late pubertal girls with obesity exhibit elevated day and night LH pulse frequency without the expected overnight decrease.[66] The latter finding seems to be related to hyperandrogenemia specifically.[69] Also of interest, LH concentration seemed to be a better predictor of free testosterone than insulin concentration in peripubertal girls with obesity.[60,70]

Recent studies indicate that serum AMH concentration, as a correlate of ovarian antral follicle number, is an important marker of PCOS risk in adolescent girls with obesity. In one study, AMH was 1.9-fold higher in adolescent girls with obesity and PCOS compared with adolescent girls with obesity alone.[71] In another study, girls with obesity born to mothers without PCOS had similar free testosterone, androstenedione, and DHEA sulfate levels compared with PCOS-d, but PCOS-d (presumed to be at higher risk for PCOS) had 2.7-fold higher AMH.[30]

HYPOTHETICAL MODEL FOR THE PUBERTAL ONTOGENY OF POLYCYSTIC OVARY SYNDROME

A hypothetical model for the pubertal ontogeny of PCOS is represented in **Fig. 1**. The model involves a genetic predisposition and possible intrauterine programming that

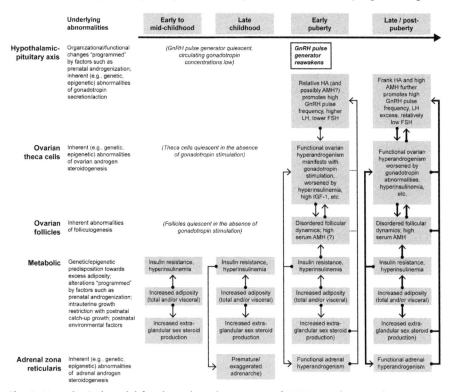

Fig. 1. Hypothetical model for the pubertal ontogeny of PCOS. HA, hyperandrogenemia.

promotes childhood hyperinsulinism, exaggerated ovarian and adrenal androgen ste-roidogenesis in response to stimulation, and postpubertal neuroendocrine dysfunc-tion. At adrenarche, corticotropin stimulates adrenals primed to secrete excess androgen; at neuroendocrine puberty, gonadotropins stimulate ovaries primed to secrete excess androgens; and both of these phenomena are enhanced by hyperin-sulinemia and elevated IGF-1 levels. Moreover, entry into neuroendocrine puberty in a hyperandrogenemic milieu impairs negative feedback at the GnRH pulse generator. This, along with elevated AMH, promotes rapid GnRH pulse frequency, increasing LH and limiting FSH release. These neuroendocrine defects further enhance hyperandro-genemia and impair ovulatory function, supporting a progression to full-blown PCOS. Although not represented in the necessarily simplistic illustration (see **Fig. 1**), numerous other factors contribute to various nodes and circuits underlying PCOS pathophysiology.

SUMMARY

It is not currently possible to diagnose presymptomatic, or even early symptomatic, PCOS in peripubertal girls. However, the study of peripubertal girls at high risk for PCOS has provided important insights into the developmental pathophysiology of PCOS. In addition to enhancing the fundamental understanding of PCOS, such research may suggest novel preventive strategies. These considerations underscore the importance of continued research into the pubertal ontogeny of PCOS.

CLINICS CARE POINTS

- Symptoms and signs of PCOS may initially manifest during puberty, but it is not currently possible to diagnose presymptomatic, or even early symptomatic, PCOS in peripubertal girls.
- Certain populations of girls are at higher risk for adolescent PCOS and should be monitored by symptoms: daughters of women with PCOS, girls with premature adrenarche, and girls with obesity.
- Definitive recommendations for prevention or early treatment in young girls at risk for PCOS are not available because of poorly understood early etiologies.
- Given that insulin resistance has been associated with the development of PCOS, healthy lifestyle (eg, diet, exercise) and maintenance of healthy weight are presumably important goals for adolescents at higher risk for PCOS; howev-er, such approaches would not address all possible etiologic mechanisms.
- For peripubertal adolescents with potential symptoms or signs of nascent PCOS, but who do not clearly meet diagnostic criteria, continued follow-up is prudent so that the diagnosis is not unnecessarily delayed.

ACKNOWLEDGMENTS

This work was supported by the Eunice Kennedy Shriver National Institute of Child Health and Human Development/National Institutes of Health through R01 HD102060 (C.M. Burt Solorzano, C.R. McCartney).

DISCLOSURE

The authors have nothing to disclose.

REFERENCES

1. McCartney CR, Marshall JC. Clinical practice. Polycystic ovary syndrome. N Engl J Med 2016;375(1):54–64.
2. Dumesic DA, Oberfield SE, Stener-Victorin E, et al. Scientific statement on the diagnostic criteria, epidemiology, pathophysiology, and molecular genetics of polycystic ovary syndrome. Endocr Rev 2015;36(5):487–525.
3. Rosenfield RL, Ehrmann DA. The pathogenesis of polycystic ovary syndrome (PCOS): the hypothesis of PCOS as functional ovarian hyperandrogenism revisited. Endocr Rev 2016;37(5):467–520.
4. Ibanez L, Oberfield SE, Witchel S, et al. An international consortium update: pathophysiology, diagnosis, and treatment of polycystic ovarian syndrome in adolescence. Horm Res Paediatr 2017;88(6):371–95.
5. Teede HJ, Misso ML, Costello MF, et al. Recommendations from the international evidence-based guideline for the assessment and management of polycystic ovary syndrome. Fertil Steril 2018;110(3):364–79.
6. Stener-Victorin E, Padmanabhan V, Walters KA, et al. Animal models to understand the etiology and pathophysiology of polycystic ovary syndrome. Endocr Rev 2020;41(4):538–76.
7. Dumont A, Robin G, Dewailly D. Anti-mullerian hormone in the pathophysiology and diagnosis of polycystic ovarian syndrome. Curr Opin Endocrinol Diabetes Obes 2018;25(6):377–84.
8. Diamanti-Kandarakis E, Dunaif A. Insulin resistance and the polycystic ovary syndrome revisited: an update on mechanisms and implications. Endocr Rev 2012; 33(6):981–1030.
9. Hiam D, Moreno-Asso A, Teede HJ, et al. The genetics of polycystic ovary syndrome: an overview of candidate gene systematic reviews and genome-wide association studies. J Clin Med 2019;8(10):1606.
10. Day F, Karaderi T, Jones MR, et al. Large-scale genome-wide meta-analysis of polycystic ovary syndrome suggests shared genetic architecture for different diagnosis criteria. PLoS Genet 2018;14(12):e1007813.
11. McCartney CR, Campbell RE. Central nervous system control in PCOS. Curr Opin Endocr Metab Res 2020;12:78–84.
12. Cimino I, Casoni F, Liu X, et al. Novel role for anti-Mullerian hormone in the regulation of GnRH neuron excitability and hormone secretion. Nat Commun 2016;7: 10055.
13. Tata B, Mimouni NEH, Barbotin AL, et al. Elevated prenatal anti-Mullerian hormone reprograms the fetus and induces polycystic ovary syndrome in adulthood. Nat Med 2018;24(6):834–46.
14. Caldwell AS, Eid S, Kay CR, et al. Haplosufficient genomic androgen receptor signaling is adequate to protect female mice from induction of polycystic ovary syndrome features by prenatal hyperandrogenization. Endocrinology 2015; 156(4):1441–52.
15. Risal S, Pei Y, Lu H, et al. Prenatal androgen exposure and transgenerational susceptibility to polycystic ovary syndrome. Nat Med 2019;25(12):1894–904.
16. Caldwell ASL, Edwards MC, Desai R, et al. Neuroendocrine androgen action is a key extraovarian mediator in the development of polycystic ovary syndrome. Proc Natl Acad Sci U S A 2017;114(16):E3334–43.
17. Sir-Petermann T, Codner E, Maliqueo M, et al. Increased anti-Mullerian hormone serum concentrations in prepubertal daughters of women with polycystic ovary syndrome. J Clin Endocrinol Metab 2006;91(8):3105–9.

18. Crisosto N, Codner E, Maliqueo M, et al. Anti-Mullerian hormone levels in peripubertal daughters of women with polycystic ovary syndrome. J Clin Endocrinol Metab 2007;92(7):2739–43.

19. Sir-Petermann T, Maliqueo M, Codner E, et al. Early metabolic derangements in daughters of women with polycystic ovary syndrome. J Clin Endocrinol Metab 2007;92(12):4637–42.

20. Sir-Petermann T, Codner E, Perez V, et al. Metabolic and reproductive features before and during puberty in daughters of women with polycystic ovary syndrome. J Clin Endocrinol Metab 2009;94(6):1923–30.

21. Maliqueo M, Sir-Petermann T, Perez V, et al. Adrenal function during childhood and puberty in daughters of women with polycystic ovary syndrome. J Clin Endocrinol Metab 2009;94(9):3282–8.

22. Crisosto N, Echiburu B, Maliqueo M, et al. Improvement of hyperandrogenism and hyperinsulinemia during pregnancy in women with polycystic ovary syndrome: possible effect in the ovarian follicular mass of their daughters. Fertil Steril 2012;97(1):218–24.

23. Maliqueo M, Galgani JE, Perez-Bravo F, et al. Relationship of serum adipocyte-derived proteins with insulin sensitivity and reproductive features in prepubertal and pubertal daughters of polycystic ovary syndrome women. Eur J Obstet Gynecol Reprod Biol 2012;161(1):56–61.

24. Sir-Petermann T, Ladron de Guevara A, Codner E, et al. Relationship between anti-Mullerian hormone (AMH) and insulin levels during different tanner stages in daughters of women with polycystic ovary syndrome. Reprod Sci 2012; 19(4):383–90.

25. Crisosto N, Ladron de Guevara A, Echiburu B, et al. Higher luteinizing hormone levels associated with antimullerian hormone in postmenarchal daughters of women with polycystic ovary syndrome. Fertil Steril 2019;111(2):381–8.

26. Torchen LC, Idkowiak J, Fogel NR, et al. Evidence for increased 5alpha-reductase activity during early childhood in daughters of women with polycystic ovary syndrome. J Clin Endocrinol Metab 2016;101(5):2069–75.

27. Trottier A, Battista MC, Geller DH, et al. Adipose tissue insulin resistance in peripubertal girls with first-degree family history of polycystic ovary syndrome. Fertil Steril 2012;98(6):1627–34.

28. Torchen LC, Fogel NR, Brickman WJ, et al. Persistent apparent pancreatic beta-cell defects in premenarchal PCOS relatives. J Clin Endocrinol Metab 2014; 99(10):3855–62.

29. Legro RS, Kunselman AR, Stetter CM, et al. Normal pubertal development in daughters of women with PCOS: a controlled study. J Clin Endocrinol Metab 2017;102(1):122–31.

30. Torchen LC, Legro RS, Dunaif A. Distinctive reproductive phenotypes in peripubertal girls at risk for polycystic ovary syndrome. J Clin Endocrinol Metab 2019;104(8):3355–61.

31. Idkowiak J, Lavery GG, Dhir V, et al. Premature adrenarche: novel lessons from early onset androgen excess. Eur J Endocrinol 2011;165(2):189–207.

32. Idkowiak J, Elhassan YS, Mannion P, et al. Causes, patterns and severity of androgen excess in 487 consecutively recruited pre- and post-pubertal children. Eur J Endocrinol 2019;180(3):213–21.

33. Ibanez L, Potau N, Virdis R, et al. Postpubertal outcome in girls diagnosed of premature pubarche during childhood: increased frequency of functional ovarian hyperandrogenism. J Clin Endocrinol Metab 1993;76(6):1599–603.

34. Ibanez L, Potau N, Zampolli M, et al. Girls diagnosed with premature pubarche show an exaggerated ovarian androgen synthesis from the early stages of puberty: evidence from gonadotropin-releasing hormone agonist testing. Fertil Steril 1997;67(5):849–55.

35. Ibanez L, Potau N, Zampolli M, et al. Hyperinsulinemia and decreased insulin-like growth factor-binding protein-1 are common features in prepubertal and pubertal girls with a history of premature pubarche. J Clin Endocrinol Metab 1997;82(7): 2283–8.

36. Ibanez L, Potau N, Chacon P, et al. Hyperinsulinaemia, dyslipaemia and cardiovascular risk in girls with a history of premature pubarche. Diabetologia 1998; 41(9):1057–63.

37. Ibanez L, Potau N, Francois I, et al. Precocious pubarche, hyperinsulinism, and ovarian hyperandrogenism in girls: relation to reduced fetal growth. J Clin Endocrinol Metab 1998;83(10):3558–62.

38. Ibanez L, Potau N, Marcos MV, et al. Adrenal hyperandrogenism in adolescent girls with a history of low birthweight and precocious pubarche. Clin Endocrinol (Oxf) 2000;53(4):523–7.

39. Ibanez L, Ong K, de Zegher F, et al. Fat distribution in non-obese girls with and without precocious pubarche: central adiposity related to insulinaemia and androgenaemia from prepuberty to postmenarche. Clin Endocrinol (Oxf) 2003; 58(3):372–9.

40. Ibanez L, de Zegher F, Potau N. Anovulation after precocious pubarche: early markers and time course in adolescence. J Clin Endocrinol Metab 1999;84(8): 2691–5.

41. Rosenfield RL, Mortensen M, Wroblewski K, et al. Determination of the source of androgen excess in functionally atypical polycystic ovary syndrome by a short dexamethasone androgen-suppression test and a low-dose ACTH test. Hum Reprod 2011;26(11):3138–46.

42. O'Reilly MW, Kempegowda P, Jenkinson C, et al. 11-Oxygenated C19 steroids are the predominant androgens in polycystic ovary syndrome. J Clin Endocrinol Metab 2017;102(3):840–8.

43. Rege J, Turcu AF, Kasa-Vubu JZ, et al. 11-Ketotestosterone is the dominant circulating bioactive androgen during normal and premature adrenarche. J Clin Endocrinol Metab 2018;103(12):4589–98.

44. Vuguin P, Linder B, Rosenfeld RG, et al. The roles of insulin sensitivity, insulin-like growth factor I (IGF-I), and IGF-binding protein-1 and -3 in the hyperandrogenism of African-American and Caribbean Hispanic girls with premature adrenarche. J Clin Endocrinol Metab 1999;84(6):2037–42.

45. Silfen ME, Manibo AM, Ferin M, et al. Elevated free IGF-I levels in prepubertal Hispanic girls with premature adrenarche: relationship with hyperandrogenism and insulin sensitivity. J Clin Endocrinol Metab 2002;87(1):398–403.

46. Silfen ME, Denburg MR, Manibo AM, et al. Early endocrine, metabolic, and sonographic characteristics of polycystic ovary syndrome (PCOS): comparison between nonobese and obese adolescents. J Clin Endocrinol Metab 2003;88(10): 4682–8.

47. Guven A, Cinaz P, Bideci A. Is premature adrenarche a risk factor for atherogenesis? Pediatr Int 2005;47(1):20–5.

48. Utriainen P, Jaaskelainen J, Romppanen J, et al. Childhood metabolic syndrome and its components in premature adrenarche. J Clin Endocrinol Metab 2007; 92(11):4282–5.

49. Ibanez L, Ong K, Valls C, et al. Metformin treatment to prevent early puberty in girls with precocious pubarche. J Clin Endocrinol Metab 2006;91(8):2888–91.
50. Ibanez L, Lopez-Bermejo A, Diaz M, et al. Metformin treatment for four years to reduce total and visceral fat in low birth weight girls with precocious pubarche. J Clin Endocrinol Metab 2008;93(5):1841–5.
51. Ibanez L, Lopez-Bermejo A, Diaz M, et al. Early metformin therapy (age 8-12 years) in girls with precocious pubarche to reduce hirsutism, androgen excess, and oligomenorrhea in adolescence. J Clin Endocrinol Metab 2011;96(8): E1262–7.
52. Anderson AD, Solorzano CM, McCartney CR. Childhood obesity and its impact on the development of adolescent PCOS. Semin Reprod Med 2014;32(3): 202–13.
53. Lim SS, Davies MJ, Norman RJ, et al. Overweight, obesity and central obesity in women with polycystic ovary syndrome: a systematic review and meta-analysis. Hum Reprod Update 2012;18(6):618–37.
54. Lizneva D, Kirubakaran R, Mykhalchenko K, et al. Phenotypes and body mass in women with polycystic ovary syndrome identified in referral versus unselected populations: systematic review and meta-analysis. Fertil Steril 2016;106(6): 1510–20.e2.
55. Christensen SB, Black MH, Smith N, et al. Prevalence of polycystic ovary syndrome in adolescents. Fertil Steril 2013;100(2):470–7.
56. Day FR, Hinds DA, Tung JY, et al. Causal mechanisms and balancing selection inferred from genetic associations with polycystic ovary syndrome. Nat Commun 2015;6:8464.
57. Brower MA, Hai Y, Jones MR, et al. Bidirectional Mendelian randomization to explore the causal relationships between body mass index and polycystic ovary syndrome. Hum Reprod 2019;34(1):127–36.
58. Reinehr T, de Sousa G, Roth CL, et al. Androgens before and after weight loss in obese children. J Clin Endocrinol Metab 2005;90(10):5588–95.
59. McCartney CR, Blank SK, Prendergast KA, et al. Obesity and sex steroid changes across puberty: evidence for marked hyperandrogenemia in pre- and early pubertal obese girls. J Clin Endocrinol Metab 2007;92(2):430–6.
60. Knudsen KL, Blank SK, Burt Solorzano C, et al. Hyperandrogenemia in obese peripubertal girls: correlates and potential etiological determinants. Obesity (Silver Spring) 2010;18(11):2118–24.
61. Kang MJ, Yang S, Hwang IT. The impact of obesity on hyperandrogenemia in Korean girls. Ann Pediatr Endocrinol Metab 2016;21(4):219–25.
62. Nokoff N, Thurston J, Hilkin A, et al. Sex differences in effects of obesity on reproductive hormones and glucose metabolism in early puberty. J Clin Endocrinol Metab 2019;104(10):4390–7.
63. Burt Solorzano CM, Helm KD, Patrie JT, et al. Increased adrenal androgens in overweight peripubertal girls. J Endocr Soc 2017;1(5):538–52.
64. de Zegher F, Reinehr T, Malpique R, et al. Reduced prenatal weight gain and/or augmented postnatal weight gain precedes polycystic ovary syndrome in adolescent girls. Obesity (Silver Spring) 2017;25(9):1486–9.
65. de Zegher F, Lopez-Bermejo A, Ibanez L. Central obesity, faster maturation, and 'PCOS' in girls. Trends Endocrinol Metab 2018;29(12):815–8.
66. McCartney CR, Prendergast KA, Blank SK, et al. Maturation of luteinizing hormone (gonadotropin-releasing hormone) secretion across puberty: evidence for altered regulation in obese peripubertal girls. J Clin Endocrinol Metab 2009; 94(1):56–66.

67. Bordini B, Littlejohn E, Rosenfield RL. Blunted sleep-related luteinizing hormone rise in healthy premenarcheal pubertal girls with elevated body mass index. J Clin Endocrinol Metab 2009;94(4):1168–75.

68. Rosenfield RL, Bordini B, Yu C. Comparison of detection of normal puberty in girls by a hormonal sleep test and a gonadotropin-releasing hormone agonist test. J Clin Endocrinol Metab 2013;98(4):1591–601.

69. Collins JS, Beller JP, Burt Solorzano C, et al. Blunted day-night changes in luteinizing hormone pulse frequency in girls with obesity: the potential role of hyperandrogenemia. J Clin Endocrinol Metab 2014;99(8):2887–96.

70. Burt Solorzano CM, Knudsen KL, Anderson AD, et al. Insulin resistance, hyperinsulinemia, and LH: relative roles in peripubertal obesity-associated hyperandrogenemia. J Clin Endocrinol Metab 2018;103(7):2571–82.

71. Kim JY, Tfayli H, Michaliszyn SF, et al. Anti-mullerian hormone in obese adolescent girls with polycystic ovary syndrome. J Adolesc Health 2017;60(3):333–9.

Fertility Issues in Polycystic Ovarian Disease

A Systematic Approach

John S. Rushing, MD[a], Nanette Santoro, MD[b],*

KEYWORDS

- PCOS • Fertility • Ovulation induction • IVF • OHSS

KEY POINTS

- Women with polycystic ovarian syndrome (PCOS) have a higher incidence of cardiometabolic challenges compared to women without the disorder. Adverse cardiometabolic indicators vary among women with PCOS, but have an indirect relationship to fertility and fertility outcomes.
- Ovulation induction is considered first-line management of infertility in women with PCOS, with letrozole superior to clomiphene.
- Women with PCOS undergoing vitro fertilization are at high risk for ovarian hyperstimulation syndrome but also have a higher live birth rate compared with controls.

HISTORY

In 1935, Dr Irving F. Stein and Dr Michael L. Leventhal were the first to describe a group of patients with the triad of hirsutism, amenorrhea, and enlarged polycystic ovaries. In their original observations, they found that several patients with amenorrhea resumed menses after an ovarian biopsy, which prompted them to create the surgical ovarian wedge procedure. They surmised that the thickened ovarian capsule prevented the follicle from releasing the egg outside of the ovary. In their original article, they discuss 7 patients with the 3 characteristics of hirsutism, amenorrhea, and enlarged polycystic ovaries who underwent bilateral ovarian wedge resection with removal of one-half to three-fourths of each ovary. All 7 patients resumed regular menses after undergoing the procedure, and 2 of the patients became pregnant.[1]

DIAGNOSTIC CRITERIA

Since Stein and Leventhal first described these patients in 1935, the syndrome has become known as polycystic ovary syndrome (PCOS). Due to the varying signs and

[a] Department of Obstetrics and Gynecology, University of Colorado, 12631 East 17th Avenue Suite B198-6, Aurora, CO 80045-2529, USA; [b] Department of Obstetrics and Gynecology, University of Colorado, 12631 East 17th Avenue Suite B198-1, Aurora, CO 80045-2529, USA
* Corresponding author.
E-mail address: nanette.santoro@cuanschutz.edu

Endocrinol Metab Clin N Am 50 (2021) 43–55
https://doi.org/10.1016/j.ecl.2020.10.004
0889-8529/21/© 2020 Elsevier Inc. All rights reserved.

symptoms patients present with, and lack of a diagnostic test, establishing criteria for the diagnosis of PCOS has been problematic. Overall, there have been 3 separate efforts[2,3] to establish diagnostic criteria for PCOS with the most commonly utilized diagnostic criterion in clinical practice being the Rotterdam criterion proposed by the European Society of Human Reproduction and Embryology and the American Society for Reproductive Medicine at a conference in Rotterdam in 2003. The investigators concluded that PCOS is a syndrome of ovarian dysfunction along with central features of hyperandrogenism and polycystic ovarian morphology and that a diagnosis of PCOS should be based on at least 2 of 3 major criteria: (1) oligo-ovulation or anovulation, (2) clinical and/or biochemical signs of hyperandrogenism, and (3) polycystic-appearing ovaries and exclusion of other etiologies (ovarian volume >10 mL^3 and/or >12 follicles between 2 mm and 9 mm in size in at least 1 ovary on ultrasound).[2] Using the Rotterdam criteria, the overall prevalence of PCOS is 10%; therefore, it is important to rule out other causes of anovulation and endocrinopathies that mimic PCOS.[4]

PATHOPHYSIOLOGY

The pathophysiology of PCOS likely is multifactorial, involving endocrine, metabolic, genetic, and environmental influences. The normal menstrual cycle is characterized by regular cyclic patterns of hormonal concentrations, whereas chronic anovulation has distorted patterns of gonadotropin and sex steroid concentrations. In women with PCOS, there is an altered pattern of gonadotropin-releasing hormone (GnRH) release that results in increased luteinizing hormone (LH) pulse frequency as well as decreased secretion of follicle-stimulating hormone (FSH), which results in impaired follicular development. The increased LH pulse frequency also allows for increased ovarian androgen production by theca cells. Women with PCOS exhibit increased circulating insulin levels, due to insulin resistance, which also contributes to hyperandrogenemia in 2 ways: (1) by stimulating ovarian androgen production and (2) by inhibiting sex hormone binding globulin by the liver. This altered pattern of gonadotropin secretion as well as chronic hyperandrogenemia and insulin resistance all contribute to ovarian dysfunction in PCOS.[5]

In women with PCOS compared with normal controls, characteristic features of the ovaries include more growing follicles, with premature growth arrest of antral follicles at 5 mm to 8 mm. This increased follicular density appears to play a role in interfering with the initiation of follicle activation and contributes to the ovarian dysfunction in PCOS. Concentrations of antimüllerian hormone (AMH), produced by granulosa cells of preantral and antral follicles, correlate with the number of these small antral follicles. The growing follicle is exposed to an atypical environment with increased LH, insulin, androgen, and AMH concentrations accompanied by insufficient FSH concentrations. These distorted interactions among the endocrine, paracrine, and autocrine factors responsible for follicular maturation contribute to ovarian dysregulation in PCOS.[6]

The role of genetics and epigenetics in PCOS increasingly is studied. Multiple studies have shown have shown increased prevalence of PCOS in siblings and parents of women with PCOS as well as hyperandrogenemia and hyperinsulinemia in first-degree relatives, suggesting a genetic susceptibility.[7,8] Genome-wide association studies have begun to identify genes involved in PCOS and currently explain approximately 10% of heritability.[9] There also are developmental programming models that suggest androgen-induced epigenetic factors and obesogenic environmental factors like the Western diet contribute to the syndrome.[10] It may take both genetic susceptibility and an obesogenic environment to fully express the phenotype.

POLYCYSTIC OVARY SYNDROME CO-CONDITIONS THAT ASSOCIATE WITH FERTILITY AND THEIR MANAGEMENT

Women with PCOS are more likely to have cardiometabolic challenges that also have an indirect relationship to their fertility and fertility outcomes. For example, women with PCOS who are of higher body mass index (BMI) have a lower likelihood of pregnancy on the basis of BMI alone.[11,12] Women with PCOS also are more likely to develop type 2 diabetes mellitus and have a more adverse cardiac risk profile than women without the disorder. In 1 sample of 122 Chicago area women with PCOS, 35% had impaired glucose tolerance and 10% had type 2 diabetes mellitus.[13] Both of these disorders have an adverse impact on subsequent pregnancy, with a higher risk of gestational diabetes mellitus (GDM) or insulin-requiring diabetes, respectively. Pregnancy-induced hypertension, present in 6.6% of normal pregnancies, is substantially more prevalent (10.8%) in women with PCOS but largely is accounted for by increased BMI.[14] More serious complications, such as preeclampsia (5.8% vs 3.6%, respectively) and life-threatening hemolysis, elevated liver enzymes, and low platelet count syndrome (4.9% vs 3.0%, respectively) also are more prevalent in pregnancies of women with PCOS compared with those without but again largely accounted for by weight. A meta-analysis that included approximately 5000 women with PCOS compared with approximately 12,000 controls found significantly greater risk in PCOS for GDM (odds ratio [OR] 3.43; 95% CI, 2.49–4.74), pregnancy-induced hypertension (OR 3.43; 95% CI, 2.49–4.74), preeclampsia (OR 2.17; 95% CI, 1.91–2.46), preterm birth (OR 1.93, 95% CI, 1.45–2.57), and cesarean section (OR 1.74; 95% CI, 1.38–2.11) compared with controls. Babies born to women with PCOS also had a marginally significant lower birth weight (weighted mean difference −0.11 g; 95% CI, −0.19 − −0.03) and higher risk of admission to a neonatal intensive care unit (OR 2.32; 95% CI, 1.40–3.85) compared with controls.[15]

Despite these challenges, the fertile life span appears to be longer in women with PCOS.[16] In a clinical sample of 500 women with PCOS compared with 500 without, pregnancy rates across the age range of 22 years to 41 years were stable in women with PCOS but declined in women with other causes for infertility. Along similar lines, using AMH levels to predict age at menopause, Minooee and colleagues[17] found that women with PCOS were likely to undergo menopause approximately 2 years later than normally ovulating women. The abundance of ovarian follicles in women with PCOS and their prolonged reproductive life span may allow them to compensate for their oligo-ovulation. In a 1966 birth cohort study from the Finnish Medical Birth Register, women with self-reported oligomenorrhea and hirsutism reported fewer children in their families but were no more likely than normo-ovulatory women to be childless.[18] Moreover, fertility may improve naturally in women with PCOS with age, because they have been reported to be more likely to become eumenorrheic in their fifth decade of life. Presumably, the loss of ovarian follicles leads to lower AMH and inhibin production, and the concomitant FSH rise drives a more normal menstrual cycle.[19]

The level of AMH has emerged as a prognostic factor for women with PCOS regardless of weight status.[20] Studies have shown that an AMH value greater than 5 ng/mL, using the second-generation AMH enzyme immunoassay, is more sensitive and specific in diagnosing PCOS than antral follicle count.[21] One of the limiting steps in determining diagnostic criteria for AMH levels in women with PCOS is the variability in AMH assays. A recent article comparing 5 different AMH immunoassays found differences in AMH values when comparing automatic and manual assays, but, when adjusting for different threshold values between the automatic and manual assays, the performance for diagnosing PCOS using the different assays was comparable.[22] At this current time, an AMH value for PCOS cutoff is not clear and there needs to be an improved standardization assays used to limit variability before AMH is incorporated into the diagnostic criteria. Women with PCOS are believed to have a congenital abundance of ovarian follicles.[23] In the early stages of follicle activation and growth, AMH is produced in these multiple follicles, which are visible on transvaginal ultrasound and lead to in higher circulating levels of the hormone. Multiple studies have converged to indicate that, based on age and BMI, an AMH level of 5 ng/mL to 10 ng/mL is associated with a high probability of PCOS.[24] AMH opposes the action of FSH in causing further growth of early activated follicles in the ovary.[25] Therefore, very high AMH levels impart an apparently paradoxic resistance to ovulation induction agents.[20] It is possible that this is a protective mechanism against promoting additional follicular development and naturally avoiding multiple gestation. In the Pregnancy in Polycystic Ovary Syndrome II study, which compared clomiphene with letrozole, the mean AMH in women who ovulated on either medication was 5.54 ng/mL compared with a mean AMH of 7.35 ng/mL among women who never achieved ovulation—despite dose escalation for both medications.[20] In this study, the antral follicle count was unrelated to the probability of ovulation. This finding implies that the amount of AMH produced per antral follicle may vary and may influence ovarian function.

There is evidence that preconceptual weight loss results in improved fertility in women with PCOS and obesity. In a comparison study of a clinical trial of 187 women with PCOS who were treated immediately with clomiphene compared with another study of 142 women with PCOS who underwent 12 weeks of weight loss and oral contraceptives prior to ovulation induction, the immediate clomiphene treatment resulted in a 10.2% live birth rate compared with 25% live birth rate in the delayed treatment with lifestyle modification (which included caloric restriction, antiobesity medication, and exercise) and oral contraceptives.[26] The mean weight loss was 6.4% in the lifestyle modification group.[27] In addition to the fertility benefit of preconception weight loss, it also may help reduce the risks, described previously, of GDM, pregnancy-induced hypertension, preeclampsia, and low-birth-weight infants. The data suggest that for women with PCOS, preconception lifestyle modification is a worthwhile intervention. As described in the Treatment of Hyperandrogenism Versus Insulin Resistance in Infertile Polycystic Ovary Syndrome (OWL PCOS) trial, the lifestyle regimen included a macronutrient balanced diet with caloric restriction (caloric deficit determined based on baseline weight and ranged from 1200 to 2000 calories per day), use of weight loss medication for women with a BMI greater than 30 kg/m^2 (sibutramine or orlistat [sibutramine was discontinued midstudy and orlistat was substituted after Food and Drug Administration approval of sibutramine was withdrawn]), coupled with a graded activity regimen with an eventual goal of 150 minutes per week. The entire lifestyle modification regimen lasted for 16 weeks; thus, women who undertake this method would postpone actively trying to conceive for approximately 4 months.[27]

OVULATION INDUCTION IN POLYCYSTIC OVARY SYNDROME

For many years, the mainstay of ovulation induction in women with PCOS was clomiphene citrate. A mixed estrogen agonist/antagonist, clomiphene has been shown to result in elevated FSH levels and an increase in LH pulse frequency in normally cycling women.[28] The increase in FSH likely is the key to its success in the treatment of women with PCOS. In the Pregnancy in Polycystic Ovary Syndrome II trial, women with well-defined PCOS had a cumulative live birth rate of 19.1% after up to 5 cycles of treatment. Most women administered clomiphene ovulate. Based on a recent individual participant meta-analysis, however, that included 3962 women with PCOS, clomiphene use resulted in an inferior live birth rate compared with the potent aromatase inhibitor, letrozole (later).

Metformin has been recommended as an agent to combat the insulin resistance in PCOS women. Metformin is effective as a diabetes preventative[29] and may facilitate weight loss. It also has been demonstrated to help regularize menstrual cycles in PCOS women.[30] Cumulative live birth rates with metformin treatment range from 19% to 37%.[31] It is not as effective a fertility treatment as clomiphene, however, and by inference, letrozole. Clomiphene and metformin were tested in a randomized clinical trial of 626 women with an outcome of live birth.[32] This was a 3-arm, multisite study that tested the efficacy of clomiphene alone, metformin alone, and metformin plus clomiphene in combination for up to 6 months for induction of ovulation. Live birth rates were 22.5% in the clomiphene alone group and 26.8% clomiphene and metformin arms of the study. Metformin alone was inferior, with a 7.2% live birth rate and a lower conception rate.

The use of metformin in combination with clomiphene has not been tested against letrozole in a randomized trial of sufficient size to examine live birth as an outcome. A recent trial of clomiphene plus low-dose (500-mg) metformin versus letrozole in 202 women with clomiphene-resistant PCOS indicated superiority of letrozole.[33] This study, however, selected for women who already had failed to conceive with clomiphene and utilized a low-dose of metformin (500 mg), which may have been inadequate to determine benefit. In the meta-analysis by Wang and colleagues,[34] women with higher baseline insulin levels derived greater benefit from the clomiphene-metformin combination compared with clomiphene alone.

More recently letrozole, a second-generation aromatase inhibitor, has been tested for its usefulness in ovulation induction and was found superior to clomiphene. A total of 750 women with PCOS were randomized to clomiphene or letrozole for up to 5 treatment cycles (**Fig. 1**). As seen in the Figure 1, 27.5% of the letrozole treated women had a live birth, which was substantially greater than the 19.1% of the clomiphene-treated women,[35] with a 3.4% versus 7.4% rate of twin pregnancies, respectively. Although letrozole overall was more effective than clomiphene in all patients, it was particularly effective in women with a higher BMI. In the individual participant meta-analysis by Wang and colleagues,[34] letrozole improved live birth rates compared with clomiphene with an relative risk of 1.43 (95% CI, 1.17–1.75). Moreover, an interaction with baseline testosterone levels was observed such that women with higher testosterone at baseline had a greater advantage with letrozole therapy for the outcome of live birth.[34] This is remarkable and somewhat counterintuitive, because letrozole is associated with an increase in circulating androgens concurrent with a rise in FSH.[36] Androgens generally are believed to not promote endometrial proliferation and even to oppose estrogen action.[37] Endometrial thickness in letrozole cycles, however, is overall greater than with clomiphene, and this may be a reason for its superiority.[38]

When standard ovulation induction medications are ineffective, exogenous gonadotropin therapy can be considered. Recombinant FSH therapy results in a high rate of ovulation, but women with PCOS are especially prone to the complications of ovarian hyperstimulation syndrome (OHSS) and higher-order multiple pregnancies. For this reason, prior to consideration of gonadotropin therapy or in vitro fertilization (IVF), laparoscopic ovarian drilling has been proposed. Approximately half of clomiphene-resistant women achieve pregnancy after laparoscopic ovarian drilling; half of women conceived without requiring any additional medication.[39] By surgically reducing the follicle burden, FSH is increased acutely, leading to ovulation. Regularity of ovulation is maintained in some women, with repeat pregnancies achieved in approximately

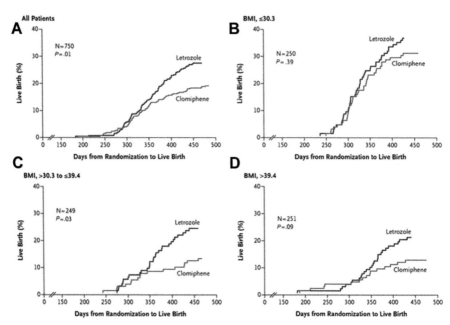

Fig. 1. Kaplan-Meier curves for live birth with clomiphene or letrozole. Live birth rates are shown according to treatment group (*A*) and according to treatment group and maternal BMI (the weight in kilograms divided by the square of the height in meters), in thirds (*B*, BMI ≤ 30.3; *C*, BMI >30.3 to ≤39.4; *D*, BMI >39.4). (*From* Legro RS, Brzyski RG, Diamond MP, et al. Letrozole versus clomiphene for infertility in the polycystic ovary syndrome. N Engl J Med 2014;371(2):119-29; with permission.)

17% of women who underwent drilling.[39] More recently, transvaginal ultrasound-assisted ovarian drilling has been recommended to avoid laparoscopy.[40]

IN VITRO FERTILIZATION IN POLYCYSTIC OVARY SYNDROME

The first live birth as a result of IVF occurred in 1978 after Robert Edwards and Patrick Steptoe[41] were able to laparoscopically retrieve an egg from a patient during a natural menstrual cycle and fertilize the egg in vitro. The developing 8-cell embryo then was transferred into the patient's uterus, which resulted in the birth of the first "test tube baby" Louise Brown.[41] Three years later, the United States had its first birth as a result of IVF.[42] Over the past 4 decades, there have been numerous advancements in the practice of IVF that have increased the success rates from in the single digits to an approximately 50% live birth rate in frozen embryo transfers from nondonor egg patients less than 35 years of age.[43] Assisted reproductive technologies (ARTs) now account for approximately 2% of all births in the United States.[44]

In its current practice, IVF is the process of stimulating the ovaries to produce multiple follicles via exogenous gonadotropins, including recombinant FSH and human menopausal gonadotropin. Patients generally receive exogenous gonadotropin stimulation for 10 days to 12 days while also using a medication to prevent ovulation. Depending on the protocol, patients can use a GnRH agonist, such as leuprolide acetate for a down-regulation approach, or a GnRH antagonist to prevent an LH surge. The patients undergoes ultrasound and laboratory monitoring on average every 2 days during stimulation to monitor estradiol levels as well as follicular growth and size. Once a patient has multiple follicles greater than 18 mm a trigger shot with human chorionic gonadotropin (HCG) and/or GnRH agonist (leuprolide acetate) is given to mimic the LH surge and stimulate oocyte maturation, keeping in mind that GnRH agonist trigger is possible only in patients receiving GnRH antagonist stimulation protocols. The eggs from the ovarian follicles then are retrieved approximately 36 hours after the trigger shot via transvaginal ultrasound with needle aspiration and subsequently fertilized in the laboratory. A resulting embryo is selected and transferred back inside the uterus typically in the blastocyst stage. IVF often is considered third-line management in women with PCOS, with ovulation induction with clomiphene or letrozole first line, followed by gonadotropin induction second line (**Table 1**).[45] Women with PCOS undergoing IVF have multiple challenges to consider, with management of an exaggerated ovarian response the most prominent.

POLYCYSTIC OVARY SYNDROME AND OVARIAN HYPERSTIMULATION SYNDROME

OHSS may occur as a result of ovarian stimulation, characterized by enlargement of the ovaries, increased vascular permeability, ascites, decreased intravascular volume, and hemoconcentration. OHSS can have varying degrees of symptoms, from mild to severe, occasionally requiring hospitalization and rare instances death.[46] Several studies have shown that patients with PCOS are at an increased risk of developing OHSS (OR 4.96; 95% CI, 3.73–6.60); this likely is a result of the increased number antral follicles in women with PCOS that results in an exaggerated follicular response and higher estradiol levels in response to induction of ovulation with gonadotropins, all risk factors for OHSS.[46–49] Due to this increased risk, several strategies have been evaluated to help prevent OHSS in patients with PCOS, including stimulation and trigger protocols as well as fresh versus frozen embryo transfers.

There are several different protocols for ovarian stimulation, and there has been debate on whether GnRH agonist versus GnRH antagonist administration should be the preferred method for ovarian stimulation of patients with PCOS. GnRH agonist protocol, also known as down-regulation protocol, includes starting a GnRH agonist, such as leuprolide acetate, in the midluteal phase of the previous menstrual cycle prior to starting recombinant FSH for ovarian stimulation in early follicular phase of the subsequent menstrual cycle. The GnRH agonist results in negative feedback of the hypothalamic-pituitary-ovarian axis, causing down-regulation of GnRH receptor activity, with resulting suppression of in LH and FSH secretion, thereby preventing LH surge and ovulation. The GnRH antagonist protocol has the same purpose as preventing early LH surge and ovulation but instead of using a GnRH agonist for down-regulation, a GnRH antagonist (ie, cetrorelix or ganirelix) is used to directly suppresses gonadotropin release. Unlike GnRH agonists, which are started in the luteal phase of

Table 1			
Fertility treatments for women with polycystic ovary syndrome			
First Line	**Second Line**	**Third Line**	**Alternatives**
Oral ovulation induction: Letrozole Clomiphene ± metformin	Gonadotropin induction	IVF	Ovarian drilling

Data from Steptoe PC, Edwards RG. Birth after the reimplantation of a human embryo. The Lancet. 1978;312(8085):366.

the prior menstrual cycle due to the initial gonadotropin surge prior to negative feedback inhibition, GnRH antagonists generally are started at approximately day 6 of IVF stimulation or if a follicle has reached 14 mm or estradiol levels of approximately 400 pg/mL. A recent meta-analysis revealed that GnRH antagonist protocol resulted in fewer severe cases of OHSS (OR 1.56; 95% CI, 0.29–8.51) while also showing no difference in clinical pregnancy rate and on-going pregnancy rate.[50] This was reaffirmed in a recent Cochrane review from 2016, showing there is moderate evidence that a GnRH antagonist protocol results in decrease OHSS.[51]

Traditionally, HCG and/or GnRH agonist administration have been the preferred methods for triggering final oocyte maturation in patients undergoing IVF, keeping in mind that a GnRH agonist only trigger is not an option in patients undergoing on agonist stimulation protocol due to the down-regulated gonadotropin receptors in the hypothalamic-pituitary axis. A systematic review from 2011 comparing GnRH agonist versus HCG for oocyte triggering in antagonist protocols showed GnRH agonist only trigger to significantly decrease the rate of OHSS (OR 0.15; 95% CI, 0.05–0.47), which is likely due to its much shorter half-life compared with HCG.[52–54] One concern with a GnRH agonist only trigger was the decreased live birth rate compared with those triggered with HCG (OR 0.47; 95% CI, 0.31–0.70), but the decrease in live birth rates was in studies using fresh autologous embryo transfers. In donor recipient cycles, there was no difference in live birth or ongoing pregnancy rates. It was surmised that the decrease in live births in fresh autologous cycles was due to an insufficient luteal phase and not related to poor embryo development from the GnRH agonist trigger.[52] Due to these findings, elective frozen embryo transfer may be the best approach in patients at high risk for OHSS such as those with PCOS.

Historically, the first embryo transfer from IVF cycles occurred on day 3 (cleavage stage) or day 5 (blastocyst stage) after oocyte retrieval and is termed, *fresh embryo transfer*. The remaining embryos were cryopreserved and stored to be thawed and transferred at a later date, termed, *frozen embryo transfer*. Small randomized and observational studies showed better outcomes in frozen embryo transfer compared with fresh transfers, which was attributed to the supraphysiologic sex steroid environment caused by ovarian stimulation that resulted in altered endometrial receptivity.[55,56] A recent multicenter randomized controlled trial evaluated fresh versus frozen embryo transfer in infertile patients with PCOS and found that frozen embryo transfer resulted in higher live birth rate (49.3% vs 42.0%, frozen vs fresh embryo transfer), for a rate ratio of 1.17 (95% CI, 1.05–1.31; $P = .004$) and lower rates of OHSS (1.3% vs 7.1%, frozen vs fresh embryo transfer), for a rate ratio of 0.19 (95% CI, 0.10–0.37; $P<.001$) but also with a higher risk of preeclampsia.[57] Another recent Cochrane review and additional randomized controlled trial evaluating fresh verses frozen embryo transfers in patients who underwent assisted reproduction showed decreased rates of OHSS in frozen embryo transfer cycles but no difference in live birth rates. This review included a variety of patients who underwent ART and was not limited to only PCOS patients.[58,59] Based on the aforementioned data, a reasonable approach to minimize OHSS while also improving live birth rates in patients with PCOS is to proceed with an antagonist protocol with GnRH agonist trigger and freeze all cycle followed by frozen embryo transfer.

IN VITRO FERTILIZATION CLINICAL OUTCOMES

According to a recent meta-analysis, women who undergo IVF secondary to PCOS have a higher live birth rate compared with controls, and there were no significant differences in rates of clinical pregnancy, multiple pregnancy, ectopic pregnancy, small for gestational age, and congenital malformations.[49] Women with PCOS, however, had significantly increased risks of miscarriage, OHSS, GDM, pregnancy-induced hypertension (PIH), large for gestational age, and preterm birth, which also has been shown by other studies.[49,60] Insulin resistance and hyperandrogenism might be potential causes of the maternal GDM, PIH, and preeclampsia.[61,62] It is important to counsel women on these risks prior to proceeding with ARTs.

SUMMARY

PCOS is a syndrome of ovarian dysfunction along with central features of hyperandrogenism and polycystic ovarian morphology; a diagnosis of PCOS should be based on at least 2 of 3 major criteria: (1) oligo-ovulation or anovulation, (2) clinical and/or biochemical signs of hyperandrogenism, and (3) polycystic-appearing ovaries. The pathophysiology of PCOS likely is multifactorial involving endocrine, metabolic, genetic, and environmental influences, and women with PCOS are more likely to have cardiometabolic challenges that also have an indirect relationship to their fertility and fertility outcomes. First-line treatment of anovulatory infertility in women with PCOS is ovulation induction with oral agents, including letrozole and clomiphene, followed by gonadotropins and lastly IVF. Letrozole has been shown superior to clomiphene citrate in ovulatory events, clinical pregnancy, and live births. Weight loss also is an effective intervention for obese women with PCOS who are infertile. Women who undergo IVF secondary to PCOS have a higher live birth rate compared with controls, and there is no significant difference in rate of clinical pregnancy, multiple pregnancy, ectopic pregnancy, small for gestational age, and congenital malformations. Women with PCOS, however, had significantly increased risks of miscarriage, OHSS, GDM, PIH, large for gestational age, and preterm birth, which also has been shown by other studies. Based on the available data, a reasonable approach to minimize OHSS, while also improving live birth rates in patients with PCOS, is to proceed with an antagonist protocol with GnRH agonist trigger and freeze all cycle followed by frozen embryo transfer.

CLINICS CARE POINTS

- PCOS is a syndrome of ovarian dysfunction with central features of hyperandrogenism and polycystic ovarian morphology; a diagnosis of PCOS should be based on at least 2 of 3 major criteria: (1) oligo-ovulation or anovulation, (2) clinical and/or biochemical signs of hyperandrogenism, and (3) polycystic-appearing ovaries.
- The level of AMH has emerged as a prognostic factor for women with PCOS, but at present, there is no agreed-upon AMH level that confirms the diagnosis of PCOS. Further standardization of AMH assays is needed before AMH can be incorporated into the diagnostic criteria for PCOS.
- First-line treatment of anovulatory infertility in women with PCOS is ovulation induction with oral agents, including letrozole and clomiphene, followed by gonadotropins and lastly IVF. Ovarian 'drilling' can be considered in the most refractory cases.
- Women with PCOS undergoing IVF are at exceptional risk for ovarian hyperstimulation syndrome, characterized by enlargement of the ovaries, increased vascular permeability, ascites, decreased intravascular volume, and hemoconcentration. Clinical caution needs to be exercised when stimulating women with PCOS with exogenous gonadotropins in order to minimize the risk of this complication.

- Based on the available data, a reasonable approach to minimize the risk of ovarian hyperstimulation while also improving live birth rates in patients with PCOS, is to proceed with an antagonist protocol with GnRH agonist trigger and freeze all embryos that are created from that cycle, followed by a cryopreserved-thawed embryo transfer in a programmed cycle.

DISCLOSURE

The authors have nothing to disclose.

REFERENCES

1. Stein IF. Amenorrhea associated with bilateral polycystic ovaries. Am J Obstet Gynecol 1935;29:181–91.
2. Rotterdam ESHRE/ASRM-Sponsored PCOS Consensus Workshop Group. Revised 2003 consensus on diagnostic criteria and long-term health risks related to polycystic ovary syndrome. Fertil Steril 2004;81(1):19–25.
3. Azziz R, Carmina E, Dewailly D, et al. The Androgen excess and PCOS Society criteria for the polycystic ovary syndrome: the complete task force report. Fertil Steril 2009;91(2):456–88.
4. Bozdag G, Mumusoglu S, Zengin D, et al. The prevalence and phenotypic features of polycystic ovary syndrome: a systematic review and meta-analysis. Hum Reprod 2016;31(12):2841–55.
5. Dumesic DA, Oberfield SE, Stener-Victorin E, et al. Scientific statement on the diagnostic criteria, epidemiology, pathophysiology, and molecular genetics of polycystic ovary syndrome. Endocr Rev 2015;36(5):487–525.
6. Witchel SF, Oberfield SE, Peña AS. Polycystic ovary syndrome: pathophysiology, presentation, and treatment with emphasis on adolescent girls. J Endocr Soc 2019;3(8):1545–73.
7. Yildiz BIO, Yarali H, Oguz H, et al. Glucose intolerance, insulin resistance, and hyperandrogenemia in first degree relatives of women with polycystic ovary syndrome. J Clin Endocrinol Metab 2003;88(5):2031–6.
8. Norman RJ, Masters S, Hague W. Hypernisulinemia is common in family members of women with polcystic ovary syndrome. Fertil Steril 1996;66(6):942–7.
9. Dunaif A. Perspectives in polycystic ovary syndrome: from hair to eternity. J Clin Endocrinol Metab 2016;101(3):759–68.
10. Carbone L, Davis BA, Fei SS, et al. Synergistic effects of hyperandrogenemia and obesogenic western-style diet on transcription and DNA methylation in visceral adipose tissue of nonhuman primates. Sci Rep 2019;9(1):1–14.
11. Gesink Law DC, Maclehose RF, Longnecker MP. Obesity and time to pregnancy. Hum Reprod 2007;22(2):414–20.
12. Jensen TK, Scheike T, Keiding N, et al. Fecundability in relation to body mass and menstrual cycle patterns. Epidemiology 1999;10(4):422–8.
13. Ehrmann DA, Barnes RB, Rosenfield RL, et al. Prevalence of impaired glucose tolerance and diabetes in women with polycystic ovary syndrome. Diabetes Care 1999;22(1):141–6.
14. Schneider D, Gonzalez JR, Yamamoto M, et al. The association of polycystic ovary syndrome and gestational hypertensive disorders in a diverse community-based cohort. J Pregnancy 2019;2019:9847057.
15. Qin JZ, Pang LH, Li MJ, et al. Obstetric complications in women with polycystic ovary syndrome: a systematic review and meta-analysis. Reprod Biol Endocrinol 2013;11:56.

16. Mellembakken JR, Berga SL, Kilen M, et al. Sustained fertility from 22 to 41 years of age in women with polycystic ovarian syndrome. Hum Reprod 2011;26(9): 2499–504.

17. Minooee S, Ramezani Tehrani F, Rahmati M, et al. Prediction of age at menopause in women with polycystic ovary syndrome. Climacteric 2018;21(1):29–34.

18. West S, Vahasarja M, Bloigu A, et al. The impact of self-reported oligo-amenorrhea and hirsutism on fertility and lifetime reproductive success: results from the Northern Finland Birth Cohort 1966. Hum Reprod 2014;29(3):628–33.

19. Elting MW, Korsen TJ, Rekers-Mombarg LT, et al. Women with polycystic ovary syndrome gain regular menstrual cycles when ageing. Hum Reprod 2000; 15(1):24–8.

20. Mumford SL, Legro RS, Diamond MP, et al. Baseline AMH level associated with ovulation following ovulation induction in women with polycystic ovary syndrome. J Clin Endocrinol Metab 2016;101(9):3288–96.

21. Dewailly D, Gronier H, Poncelet E, et al. Diagnosis of polycystic ovary syndrome (PCOS): revisiting the threshold values of follicle count on ultrasound and of the serum AMH level for the definition of polycystic ovaries. Hum Reprod 2011; 26(11):3123–9.

22. Pigny P, Gorisse E, Ghulam A, et al. Comparative assessment of five serum anti-müllerian hormone assays for the diagnosis of polycystic ovary syndrome. Fertil Steril 2016;105(4):1063–9.e3.

23. Welt CK, Carmina E. Lifecycle of polycystic ovary syndrome (PCOS): from in utero to menopause. J Clin Endocrinol Metab 2013;98(12):4629–38.

24. Quinn MM, Kao CN, Ahmad AK, et al. Age-stratified thresholds of anti-Mullerian hormone improve prediction of polycystic ovary syndrome over a population-based threshold. Clin Endocrinol (Oxf) 2017;87(6):733–40.

25. Durlinger AL, Gruijters MJ, Kramer P, et al. Anti-Mullerian hormone attenuates the effects of FSH on follicle development in the mouse ovary. Endocrinology 2001; 142(11):4891–9.

26. Legro RS, Dodson WC, Kunselman AR, et al. Benefit of delayed fertility therapy with preconception weight loss over immediate therapy in obese women with PCOS. J Clin Endocrinol Metab 2016;101(7):2658–66.

27. Legro RS, Dodson WC, Kris-Etherton PM, et al. Randomized controlled trial of preconception interventions in infertile women with polycystic ovary syndrome. J Clin Endocrinol Metab 2015;100(11):4048–58.

28. Kettel LM, Roseff SJ, Berga SL, et al. Hypothalamic-pituiary-ovarina response to clomiphene citrate in women with polycystic ovary syndrome. Fertil Steril 1993; 59(3):532–8.

29. Knowler WC, Barrett-Connor E, Fowler SE, et al. Reduction in the incidence of type 2 diabetes with lifestyle intervention or metformin. N Engl J Med 2002; 346(6):393–403.

30. Yang PK, Hsu CY, Chen MJ, et al. The efficacy of 24-month metformin for improving menses, hormones, and metabolic profiles in polycystic ovary syndrome. J Clin Endocrinol Metab 2018;103(3):890–9.

31. Sharpe A, Morley LC, Tang T, et al. Metformin for ovulation induction (excluding gonadotrophins) in women with polycystic ovary syndrome. Cochrane Database Syst Rev 2019;(12):CD013505.

32. Legro RS, Barnhart HX, Schlaff WD, et al. Clomiphene, metformin, or both for infertility in the polycystic ovary syndrome. N Engl J Med 2007;356(6):551–66.

33. Rezk M, Shaheen AE, Saif El-Nasr I. Clomiphene citrate combined with metformin versus letrozole for induction of ovulation in clomiphene-resistant polycystic ovary syndrome: a randomized clinical trial. Gynecol Endocrinol 2018;34(4):298–300.
34. Wang R, Li W, Bordewijk EM, et al. First-line ovulation induction for polycystic ovary syndrome: an individual participant data meta-analysis. Hum Reprod Update 2019;25(6):717–32.
35. Legro RS, Brzyski RG, Diamond MP, et al. Letrozole versus clomiphene for infertility in the polycystic ovary syndrome. N Engl J Med 2014;371(2):119–29.
36. Kucherov A, Polotsky AJ, Menke M, et al. Aromatase inhibition causes increased amplitude, but not frequency, of hypothalamic-pituitary output in normal women. Fertil Steril 2011;95(6):2063–6.
37. Zang H, Sahlin L, Masironi B, et al. Effects of testosterone treatment on endometrial proliferation in postmenopausal women. J Clin Endocrinol Metab 2007;92(6):2169–75.
38. Wang L, Wen X, Lv S, et al. Comparison of endometrial receptivity of clomiphene citrate versus letrozole in women with polycystic ovary syndrome: a randomized controlled study. Gynecol Endocrinol 2019;35(10):862–5.
39. Debras E, Fernandez H, Neveu ME, et al. Ovarian drilling in polycystic ovary syndrome: long term pregnancy rate. Eur J Obstet Gynecol Reprod Biol X 2019;4:100093.
40. Zhang J, Tang L, Kong L, et al. Ultrasound-guided transvaginal ovarian needle drilling for clomiphene-resistant polycystic ovarian syndrome in subfertile women. Cochrane Database Syst Rev 2019;(7):CD008583.
41. Steptoe PC, Edwards RG. Birth after the reimplantation of a human embryo. Lancet 1978;312(8085):366.
42. Jones HWIVF Jr. past and future. Reprod Biomed Online 2003;6(3):375–81.
43. CDC; American Society for Reproductive Medicine; Society for Assisted Reproductive Technology. 2015 assisted reproductive technology fertility clinic success rates report. Atlanta, GA: US Department of Health and Human Services; 2017.
44. Sunderam S, Kissin DM, Zhang Y, et al. Assisted Reproductive Technology Surveillance-United States, 2016. MMWR Surveill Summ 2019;68(4):1–23.
45. Group TTEA-SPCW. Consensus on infertility treatment related to polycystic ovary syndrome. Hum Reprod 2008;23(3):462–77.
46. Practice Committee of the American Society for Reproductive Medicine. Prevention and treatment of moderate and severe ovarian hyperstimulation syndrome: a guideline. Fertil Steril 2016;106(7):1634–47.
47. Enskog A, Henriksson M, Unander M, et al. Prospective study of the clinical and laboratory parameters of patients in whom ovarian hyperstimulation syndrome developed during controlled ovarian hyperstimulation for in vitro fertilization. Fertil Steril 1999;71(5):808–14.
48. Swanton A, Storey L, McVeigh E, et al. IVF outcome in women with PCOS, PCO and normal ovarian morphology. Eur J Obstet Gynecol Reprod Biol 2010;149(1):68–71.
49. Sha T, Wang X, Cheng W, et al. A meta-analysis of pregnancy-related outcomes and complications in women with polycystic ovary syndrome undergoing in vitro fertilization. Reprod Biomed Online 2019;39(2):281–93.
50. Lin H, Li Y, Li L, et al. Is a GnRH antagonist protocol better in PCOS patients? A meta-analysis of RCTs. PLoS One 2014;9(3):e91796.
51. Al-Inany HG, Youssef MA, Ayeleke RO, et al. Gonadotrophin-releasing hormone antagonists for assisted reproductive technology. Cochrane Database Syst Rev 2016;(4):CD001750.

52. Youssef MA, Van der Veen F, Al-Inany HG, et al. Gonadotropin-releasing hormone agonist versus HCG for oocyte triggering in antagonist assisted reproductive technology cycles. Cochrane Database Syst Rev 2011;(1):CD008046.

53. Delvigne A. Epidemiology of OHSS. Reprod Biomed Online 2009;19(1):8–13.

54. Abbara A, Islam R, Clarke S, et al. Clinical parameters of ovarian hyperstimulation syndrome following different hormonal triggers of oocyte maturation in IVF treatment. Clin Endocrinol 2018;88(6):920–7.

55. Kalra SK, Ratcliffe SJ, Milman L, et al. Perinatal morbidity after in vitro fertilization is lower with frozen embryo transfer. Fertil Steril 2011;95(2):548–53.

56. Shapiro BS, Daneshmand ST, Garner FC, et al. Evidence of impaired endometrial receptivity after ovarian stimulation for in vitro fertilization: a prospective randomized trial comparing fresh and frozen–thawed embryo transfer in normal responders. Fertil Steril 2011;96(2):344–8.

57. Chen Z-J, Shi Y, Sun Y, et al. Fresh versus frozen embryos for infertility in the polycystic ovary syndrome. N Engl J Med 2016;375:523–33.

58. Wong KM, van Wely M, Mol F, et al. Fresh versus frozen embryo transfers in assisted reproduction. Cochrane Database Syst Rev 2017;(3):CD011184.

59. Shi Y, Sun Y, Hao C, et al. Transfer of fresh versus frozen embryos in ovulatory women. N Engl J Med 2018;378(2):126–36.

60. Sterling L, Liu J, Okun N, et al. Pregnancy outcomes in women with polycystic ovary syndrome undergoing in vitro fertilization. Fertil Steril 2016;105(3):791–7.e2.

61. Toulis KA, Goulis DG, Kolibianakis EM, et al. Risk of gestational diabetes mellitus in women with polycystic ovary syndrome: a systematic review and a meta-analysis. Fertil Steril 2009;92(2):667–77.

62. Chen M-J, Yang W-S, Yang J-H, et al. Relationship between androgen levels and blood pressure in young women with polycystic ovary syndrome. Hypertension 2007;49(6):1442–7.

Management of Women with Polycystic Ovary Syndrome During Pregnancy

Amy M. Valent, DO[a],*, Linda A. Barbour, MD, MSPH[b,c]

KEYWORDS

- Polycystic ovary syndrome • Pregnancy complications • Perinatal management
- Metformin

KEY POINTS

- Polycystic ovary syndrome (PCOS) is associated with adverse pregnancy outcomes, independent of high-risk, PCOS-related conditions.
- The preconception period is the best opportunity to discuss pregnancy-related complications, preventative screening, and safe treatments during pregnancy and to implement nutritional and lifestyle behaviors to improve oocyte quality and potentially pregnancy outcomes.
- Metformin treatment is not recommended for women with PCOS during pregnancy because it has not been demonstrated to improve perinatal outcomes. It is often recommended for PCOS outside of pregnancy due to its favorable metabolic outcomes in women with PCOS. Therefore, because metformin is not associated with an increased risk for teratogenicity or breastfeeding, it may be continued through the first trimester and immediately resumed postpartum.

INTRODUCTION

Polycystic ovarian syndrome (PCOS) affects approximately 1 in 10 reproductive age women of all races and ethnicities.[1,2] However, the phenotypic heterogeneity among women with PCOS variably affect pregnancy outcomes. Women with PCOS may have challenges conceiving secondary to the effects of obesity, metabolic dysfunction including insulin resistance (IR), inflammation, or endocrine abnormalities. These conditions influence ovulatory function, endometrial receptivity, and oocyte quality.[3] The phenotypic variability of PCOS and differences in diagnostic criteria from adolescence

[a] Department of Obstetrics and Gynecology, Oregon Health and Science University, 3181 Southwest Sam Jackson Park Road, Mail Location L-458, Portland, OR 97239, USA; [b] Department of Medicine, University of Colorado Anschutz Medical Campus, 12801 East 17th Avenue, RC1 South Room 7103, Aurora, CO 80045, USA; [c] Department of Obstetrics and Gynecology, University of Colorado Anschutz Medical Campus, 12801 East 17th Avenue, RC1 South Room 7103, Aurora, CO 80045, USA
* Corresponding author.
E-mail address: valent@ohsu.edu

Endocrinol Metab Clin N Am 50 (2021) 57–69
https://doi.org/10.1016/j.ecl.2020.10.005   endo.theclinics.com
0889-8529/21/© 2020 Elsevier Inc. All rights reserved.

to adulthood have contributed to the research, intervention, and clinical management challenges for this condition.[1,4]

Pregnant women with PCOS have increased risks for adverse pregnancy outcomes, independent of subfertility and use of assisted reproductive technology (ART).[5] Adverse perinatal outcomes include early pregnancy loss, gestational diabetes mellitus (GDM), hypertensive spectrum disorder (ie, gestational hypertension [HTN] and preeclampsia), small- and large-for-gestational-age infants (SGA, LGA), preterm birth, and cesarean deliveries.[6–8] The pathobiology of these adverse perinatal outcomes among women with PCOS is debated. The metabolic, genetic, clinical, and biochemical characteristics of PCOS contribute to an altered intrauterine environment, increased risks for pregnancy complications, and long-term fetal developmental programming risks observed in this higher risk population.

Despite the higher rates of adverse pregnancy outcomes associated with PCOS, there is no consensus on perinatal guidelines specific to the management of PCOS in pregnancy. A paucity of studies with poorly characterized metabolic phenotypes have been done using pharmacologic and surveillance measures to reduce perinatal complications among women with PCOS. Increased surveillance and clinical management strategies during pregnancy have been directed from PCOS-related conditions and characteristics.[9,10]

PERINATAL OUTCOMES

PCOS is complicated by phenotypic heterogeneity, different diagnostic criteria, and variable chronic health conditions that an individual may have entering pregnancy, which challenges the development of evidenced-based strategies to improve pregnancy outcomes. PCOS-related comorbidities include overweight/obesity, IR, dyslipidemia, low-grade chronic inflammation, mental health disorders, and HTN.[11,12] Even after adjusting for these high-risk factors, PCOS is associated with an increased risk of adverse perinatal outcomes (**Fig. 1**), but the effect of the different PCOS phenotypes on these adverse outcomes are conflicting.[13,14]

Women with PCOS who undergo in vitro fertilization (IVF) have similar clinical pregnancy rates as other women who undergo IVF for other infertility causes. In a recent meta-analysis, among women who underwent IVF, PCOS was associated with higher rates of miscarriage (odds ratio [OR] 1.52; 95% confidence interval [CI] 1.04–2.22, $I^2 = 21.4\%$), ovarian hyperstimulation syndrome (OR 4.62; 95% CI 3.20–6.68; $I^2 = 0\%$), GDM (OR 2.67; 95% CI 1.43–4.98; I = 61%), gestational HTN (OR 2.06; 95% CI 1.45–2.91; I = 28.3%), LGA (OR 2.10; 95% CI 1.01–4.37; I = 65.7%), and preterm birth ([PTB]; OR 1.60; 95% CI 1.25–2.04) compared with IVF performed for other causes of infertility.[5] The review was limited by varying degrees of heterogeneity between the studies and the limited number of prospective studies included in the analysis but underscore the significant risks associated with PCOS among this higher risk IVF population.

The most common pregnancy complications reported among women with PCOS are GDM (OR 2.78–3.58) and hypertensive spectrum disorder (OR 2.46–3.43), which are significantly increased, independent of age, fertility treatment, obesity status, or other confounding demographic factors.[7,8,15,16] A significant number of these women meet criteria for metabolic syndrome; research models have suggested preconception or early pregnancy measures of sex-hormone binding globulin, afamin, androstenedione, fasting glucose and triglycerides, and IR as potential predictors of GDM among the PCOS population. These metabolic markers are in addition to known risk factors such as age, obesity, prediabetes, family history of diabetes, and history

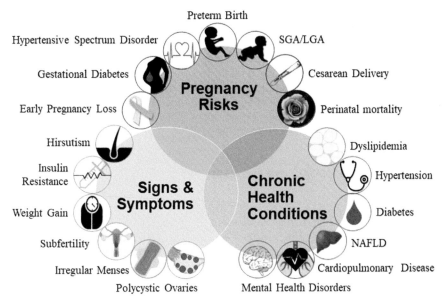

Hypertensive Spectrum Disorder

Preterm Birth

SGA/LGA

Gestational Diabetes

Pregnancy Risks

Cesarean Delivery

Early Pregnancy Loss

Perinatal mortality

Hirsutism

Dyslipidemia

Insulin Resistance

Signs & Symptoms

Chronic Health Conditions

Hypertension

Weight Gain

Diabetes

Subfertility

NAFLD

Irregular Menses

Cardiopulmonary Disease

Polycystic Ovaries

Mental Health Disorders

Fig. 1. PCOS is a complex disorder that is associated with increased risks for perinatal complications and significant chronic health conditions. NAFLD, nonalcoholic fatty liver; SGA/LGA, small-/large-for-gestational-age.

of GDM.[17–20] However, prospective studies are needed to determine the efficacy of these markers in predicting GDM among women with PCOS.

The association of PCOS with adverse neonatal outcomes is inconsistent. In the most recent meta-analyses, PCOS was associated with an increase in the risk for PTB (OR 1.52–1.93).[5,7,16] However, the studies included in the analyses did not distinguish spontaneous versus indicated PTB, which is important for the utility of available preventative interventions for a history of spontaneous PTB. Studies have reported an increased risk for both SGA and LGA among women with PCOS but only when considering prospective studies and within specific populations.[5,7] Opposite growth outcomes may suggest different underlying comorbidities known to affect growth, including IR, prediabetes, dyslipidemia, hypertensive disorders, obesity, obstructive sleep apnea (OSA), and over-/undernutrition. Neonates born to mothers with PCOS have higher rates of neonatal intensive care unit (NICU) admissions (OR 1.74–2.31) and perinatal mortality (OR 1.83–3.07).[7,15,16]

PLACENTAL CONTRIBUTIONS IN ADVERSE OUTCOMES

The placenta is the largest endocrine organ during pregnancy, communicating with both the fetus and the mother to ensure normal fetal development and growth. The placenta serves as a mediator of pregnancy complications, neonatal outcomes, and developmental programming of the offspring.[21] Human studies suggest higher prevalence of placental infarctions, villitis, and villous immaturity even after adjusting for significant demographic and pregnancy complications associated with PCOS during pregnancy.[22] The variable PCOS phenotype and the significant maternal and neonatal morbidities associated with PCOS have contributed to the challenges and paucity of studies focused on placental dysfunction and contributions to adverse outcomes.

Animal models of maternal hyperandrogenism, IR, and overnutrition demonstrate altered placental angiogenesis, nutrient sensing and transport, and vascular blood flow.[23,24]

Variations in fetoplacental development may lead to changes in fetal nutrient and oxygen supply that influence early growth and development.[25] Offspring born to women with PCOS are associated with increased risks for higher childhood body mass index (BMI), abnormal cardiometabolic markers, and neurodevelopmental disorders.[26] The genetic and epigenetic contributions of PCOS, PCOS-related comorbidities, and adverse pregnancy conditions (ie, GDM, SGA, LGA, and preeclampsia) affect the intrauterine environment and long-term offspring health (**Fig. 2**).

PERICONCEPTION, PRENATAL, AND POSTPARTUM EVALUATION AND MANAGEMENT
Periconception

Individuals with PCOS have multiple factors that are associated with increased perinatal complications.[27] Pregnancy is often a motivating period for individuals and families; optimizing health before pregnancy may improve pregnancy outcomes and maternal lifelong health. The preconception period provides a window of opportunity where pregnancy-related complications can be discussed, preventative screening and safe treatments during pregnancy can be initiated, and nutritional and lifestyle behaviors can be optimized to improve oocyte quality and potentially pregnancy outcomes.[28,29]

Prepregnancy BMI is strongly associated with adverse perinatal outcomes and incrementally increases the risk for preeclampsia, GDM, indicated preterm delivery, and macrosomia.[30] Lifestyle interventions incorporating high-quality nutrition, physical activity, and behavioral strategies should be advised before pregnancy as the primary approach to aid in losing weight and improving health.[31] Studies have demonstrated improved fecundity and live birth rates among modest weight-loss (5%–10% of initial body weight) and healthy lifestyle interventions in the subfertile

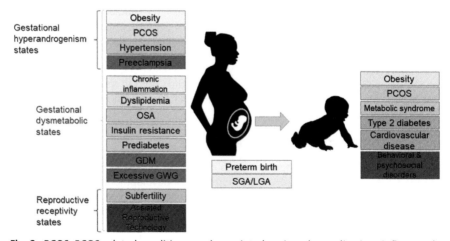

Fig. 2. PCOS, PCOS-related conditions, and associated perinatal complications influence the intrauterine environment, leading to the developmental programming of the offspring for long-term, chronic health conditions. GDM, gestational diabetes; SGA/LGA, small-/large-for-gestational-age.

PCOS population, but trials showing a benefit from a weight-loss intervention prepregnancy to reduce pregnancy-related complications are currently lacking.[32] Antiobesity medications are not recommended during pregnancy, and women should be advised to discontinue and implement other strategies before pregnancy.[33] Although bariatric surgery has been shown to decrease rates of GDM, hypertensive disorders, and macrosomia, it has associated risks with potential postsurgical complications, fetal growth restriction, and nutritional challenges that need to be considered.[34] Among women who undergo bariatric surgery, pregnancy should be avoided within 1 year of the operation or weight stabilization. Bariatric surgery often improves IR, impaired glucose tolerance (IGT), hyperlipidemia, and sleep-disordered breathing, but as an intervention to improve conception rates or pregnancy-related complications among women with PCOS is considered investigational.

PCOS is also associated with an increased risk of depression, anxiety, bipolar disorder, eating disorders, and obsessive compulsive disorder, particularly among individuals with weight concerns or subfertility.[35,36] Routine screening for depression, anxiety, and other mental health disorders are recommended upon diagnosis of PCOS and if negative to screen again among those with high-risk factors such as obesity, diabetes, pregnancy, postpartum, or family history of mental health disorders.[35] Individuals found to have positive mental health screens should be offered or referred for cognitive behavioral therapy and/or interpersonal therapy.[37]

IR, hyperinsulinemia, and IGT are common features observed among individuals with PCOS that may present even during adolescence. Because of the increased risk for GDM, women are recommended to be screened for diabetes and cardiovascular risk factors (ie, obesity, dyslipidemia, HTN, and nicotine use) before conception.[9,10] International guidelines have recommended a 75-g oral glucose tolerance test (OGTT) to be offered in all women with PCOS when planning pregnancy or seeking fertility treatment.[38] If not performed preconception, overweight/obese individuals (BMI $\geq$25 kg/m^2 or $\geq$23 kg/m^2 in Asian Americans) with PCOS are considered a high-risk population and should be screened early in gestation for preexisting diabetes/prediabetes using an OGTT and again at 24 to 28 weeks if early testing results are normal.[10,39] Women taking metformin should discontinue the medication for at least 3 to 5 days before OGTT.

IR and obesity are strongly associated with sleep-breathing disorders. OSA increases the risk for GDM and preeclampsia 2- to 3-fold in addition to more rare maternal outcomes such as cardiomyopathy, pulmonary edema, and mortality.[40] Even mild OSA, shown to occur in up to two-thirds of pregnant women with obesity, is correlated with mild hyperglycemia and higher free fatty acids, cortisol, and hepatic IR.[41] Therefore, women with PCOS should be screened for symptoms related to sleep-breathing disorders preconception and throughout pregnancy.[42]

Prenatal

Women with PCOS have higher risks for adverse pregnancy outcomes and are recommended to have closer surveillance during the prenatal and postpartum period. Even after adjusting for significant confounders, individuals with PCOS have up to a 2-fold higher risk for hypertensive spectrum disorder and GDM.[8] However, there are no specific guidelines for antenatal fetal surveillance or ultrasound assessments for PCOS. Recommendations for this population is driven by the high-risk characteristics that women with PCOS commonly have (ie, ART, obesity, GDM, and HTN). Therefore, individualized fetal surveillance and perinatal management is recommended.

Metformin use during pregnancy among women with polycystic ovary syndrome
Metformin has been widely used in women with PCOS for induction ovulation, to improve insulin sensitivity and treat prediabetes in women planning to conceive. It readily crosses the placenta, but studies do not demonstrate an associated teratogenic risk with short-term use of metformin during pregnancy.[43,44] Metformin has not been shown by most of the randomized controlled trials (RCTs) to improve pregnancy outcomes, including miscarriage, PTB, excess gestational weight gain (GWG), GDM, LGA, or preeclampsia.[45] Moreover, concerns about potential long-term offspring risks due to its pleiotropic effects and concentration into fetal mitochondria dampen the enthusiasm for its use in women with PCOS during pregnancy.[46]

Although some observational trials and meta-analyses have suggested that metformin may decrease early pregnancy loss and preterm delivery,[47] the American Society for Reproductive Medicine published guidelines on the role of metformin for ovulation induction in PCOS and concluded insufficient evidence that metformin alone increases live birth rates or decreases miscarriage. Further, discontinuing metformin once pregnancy is confirmed does not affect the rate of miscarriage.[48]

The Preg-Met study was an RCT among women with PCOS (Rotterdam criteria) who were randomized to 1700 to 2000 mg metformin versus placebo at 5 to 12 weeks of pregnancy in 11 centers in Norway.[49] In both Preg-Met and Preg-Met 2, metformin did not statistically reduce GDM, preeclampsia, preterm birth, cesarean delivery, birthweight, or macrosomia (defined as >4500g).[49,50] Similarly, a Cochrane review and meta-analysis, which included RCTs of high-risk women with PCOS, obesity, or IR who were treated with metformin periconception or before 20 weeks gestation, did not improve GDM risk (risk ratio 1.03; 95% CI 0.85–1.24) compared with placebo.[45–47,51,52] Metformin's ability to decrease hypertensive spectrum disorder during pregnancy remains unclear,[53] but there are no adequately powered RCTs in PCOS to evaluate this endpoint.[54] Although lower GWG was achieved with metformin use during pregnancy, approximately 50% of the participants in the Preg-Met study who were followed for an average of 7.7 (5–11) years demonstrated no difference in subsequent weight gain, BMI, waist/hip ratio, blood pressure, body composition, lipids, glucose, insulin levels, or metabolic syndrome at follow-up compared with the referent/placebo group.[49,50,55]

The available data are insufficient to support metformin use to prevent miscarriage or PTB. Although women with PCOS, particularly with IR prepregnancy, have higher rates of GDM, current evidence does not support using metformin in women with PCOS or obesity to prevent GDM, preeclampsia, or LGA. Long-term use of metformin seems to be effective at reducing β-cell demand and progression of GDM to type 2 diabetes mellitus (T2DM).[56,57] However, it is unlikely that the short-term, marked IR of pregnancy, and the demand for a 2-fold increase in insulin secretion can be significantly mitigated by metformin.

Pleiotropic effects of metformin on fetoplacental tissues and potential for long-term metabolic offspring consequences
Metformin is transported by organic cation transporters into mitochondrial membranes that are present abundantly in both the fetus and placenta. The embryo has few, and relatively immature, mitochondria due to low rates of aerobic metabolism and expresses very low levels of organic cation transporters. Therefore, it is considered safe in the first trimester and can be continued until organogenesis is completed. However, fetal levels of metformin have been shown to be at least as high as maternal levels at time of delivery (make sure the reader knows this is not referring to first trimester).[58] Fetal metabolic health could be affected by metformin's cellular effects,

which include impairment of glycolysis, tricarboxylic acid cycle, histone acetylation, and one-carbon metabolism; inhibition of mitochondrial activity, mTOR, and cell cycle proliferation; suppression of protein synthesis; or induction of epigenetic modifications.[43,59,60]

Offspring of women with PCOS randomized to metformin versus placebo, followed-up through approximately 10 years of life, suggest metformin-exposed offspring have higher risks for increased weight, BMI z-scores, and waist circumference without a difference in mean IQ function.[61–65] These findings are consistent with a 7- to 9-year follow-up of the offspring among women with GDM randomized to metformin versus placebo in the Metformin in Gestation (MiG) RCT.[66] A meta-analysis of all of the offspring cohorts from the MiG trial concluded that neonates born to metformin-treated mothers had lower birth weights, LGA, and macrosomia rates compared with mothers treated with insulin with no difference in SGA. However, metformin-exposed children seem to have accelerated postnatal growth, resulting in heavier infants and higher BMI by midchildhood.[67] The PCOS and GDM offspring studies were limited by relatively small follow-up populations from the original cohorts. A systematic review and meta-analysis of GDM or PCOS RCTs (778 children) of mothers randomized to metformin versus insulin or placebo concluded that prenatal metformin was associated with increased offspring weight but not height or BMI during childhood.[68] Recently, the Metformin in Type 2 Diabetes RCT (MiTY) was completed, which randomized 502 women with T2DM on insulin to metformin or placebo in 25 centers in Canada and 4 in Australia and included ~17% of women with PCOS (MiTy). Although there were no differences between the groups in the primary composite outcome (pregnancy loss, preterm birth [<37 weeks' gestation], birth injury, moderate or severe respiratory distress syndrome, neonatal hypoglycemia, and NICU admission lasting greater than 24 hours) or hypertensive disorders in pregnancy, women randomized to metformin had lower insulin requirements, hemoglobin A1C (mean 5.9 vs 6.1), gestational weight gain, LGA, macrosomia, and C-section but an almost 2-fold increase in SGA.[69] The participating institutions anticipate following the children long term to determine the long-term implications of metformin exposure during pregnancy, particularly among offspring born SGA.

Metformin has the potential to inhibit mitochondrial activity and result in relative nutrient restriction that could potentially affect function, growth, or differentiation of fetal or placental tissues. It is plausible that mild nutrient restriction prenatally followed by nutrient excess in childhood could predispose an increased obesity risk. Further studies on metformin's effects on the placenta and postnatal metabolic vulnerability are needed to address these gaps.[43,70] However, given that metformin readily crosses the placenta and the insufficient data to support improvements on short-term pregnancy outcomes in women with PCOS, its use beyond the first trimester should be limited to special circumstances with a discussion of potential offspring risks or to research studies designed to examine longitudinal perinatal and childhood outcomes.

Postpartum

The postpartum period is an opportunity for preconception and long-term health optimization. Unfortunately, less than 50% of pregnant individuals return for postpartum care. The American College of Obstetricians and Gynecologists recently emphasized the importance of the postpartum period in optimizing the health of women, infants, and families. Postpartum care should be viewed as an ongoing process with anticipatory guidance beginning in the prenatal period, individualizing a comprehensive care plan to include mood and overall well-being, infant care and feeding, contraception, birth spacing, sleep, delivery recovery, chronic health management, and goals for long-term health maintenance.[71] One in seven pregnancies are complicated by post-partum depression,[72] which is associated with significant maternal and neonatal morbidity and mortality. PCOS is a high-risk condition, but studies are inconclusive on whether the prevalence of postpartum depression is increased in this population.[73] However, screening for depression and anxiety should be performed through the first year postpartum.[37]

The limited data on PCOS and breastfeeding suggest overall lower breastfeeding success among PCOS, but these studies were confounded by other factors associated with decreased breastfeeding success (ie, BMI and pregnancy complications) and did not account for breastfeeding intention.[74] Although PCOS is commonly associated with biologically plausible physiologic and psychological causes of breastfeeding challenges, such as IR, hyperandrogenism effects on prolactin, and breast tissue transformation; higher BMI is a stronger risk factor for lower breastfeeding rates than PCOS alone.[75] The benefits of breastfeeding intensity and duration with future maternal and offspring health risks have not been specifically studied in PCOS. However, women who develop GDM and breastfeed for at least 6 months reduce their risk for T2DM and the long-term risk to their offspring for childhood obesity.[76,77]

One of the strongest risk factors for later obesity, metabolic disease, and T2DM is postpartum weight retention.[78] Targeted efforts to facilitate weight loss are critical for both risk reduction in the subsequent pregnancy and long-term maternal health. The Diabetes Prevention Program and the Diabetes Prevention Program Outcomes Study have demonstrated intensive lifestyle or metformin are highly effective in reducing the progression of diabetes and cost-savings among individuals at high risk for T2DM.[56,79,80] Encouraging the continuation of healthy lifestyle interventions and resuming or initiating metformin in the postpartum period are important for preventing the progression of metabolic dysfunction and T2DM. Metformin can be immediately resumed postpartum. Although the data are limited, metformin excretion in breastmilk seems to be very low at less than 1% of the mother's weight-adjusted dose with no reports of infant hypoglycemia.[81]

PCOS is associated with multiple health factors and adverse pregnancy outcomes that can challenge the transition from pregnancy to parenthood and long-term chronic health disease management. Focusing on maternal health during this "fourth trimester" can help women with PCOS navigate through these transitions, coordinate ongoing care of chronic conditions, decrease maternal morbidity and mortality, and importantly optimize long-term family health.

CLINICAL CARE POINTS

- Women with PCOS should be informed of their increased pregnancy risks, including early pregnancy loss, GDM, hypertensive spectrum disorder, SGA, LGA, PTB, and cesarean deliveries.
- Preconception health optimization to screen for mood disorders, diabetes, and cardiopulmonary risk factors with the implementation of lifestyle interventions or specific therapies is strongly recommended. Prospective, preconception intervention studies are needed to determine efficacy of reducing adverse pregnancy outcomes.
- Offspring of women with PCOS have higher rates of increased BMI, abnormal cardiometabolic markers, and neurodevelopmental disorders. Further studies are needed to understand the genetic and epigenetic contributions of PCOS, PCOS-related comorbidities, placenta's role in nutrient availability, and influence of medications that may affect the long-term offspring health.

- Pregnant women with PCOS are recommended to have increased surveillance and individualized care plans based on PCOS-related conditions and known risk factors that increase the risk for adverse perinatal outcomes. Prospective studies using consistent diagnostic criteria and metabolically phenotyped participants are necessary to better understand PCOS-specific contributions to adverse perinatal outcomes.
- Metformin is not recommended to be continued beyond the first trimester to improve perinatal outcomes, but it can be immediately restarted after delivery. More longitudinal and mechanistic studies are needed to determine whether metformin treatment during pregnancy seems to adversely affect childhood obesity and future health risks.
- Postpartum is an important transitional period, and a paucity of studies specifically address postpartum challenges among women with PCOS. Women are recommended to have an individualized comprehensive care plan that begins prenatally and followed through the first year postpartum to optimize transitions to parenthood, long-term conditions, and preconception health for future pregnancies.

DISCLOSURE

The authors have no conflicts of interest to disclose.

REFERENCES

1. Fauser BC, Tarlatzis BC, Rebar RW, et al. Consensus on women's health aspects of polycystic ovary syndrome (PCOS): the Amsterdam ESHRE/ASRM-Sponsored 3rd PCOS Consensus Workshop Group. Fertil Steril 2012;97(1):28–38.e25.
2. Wolf WM, Wattick RA, Kinkade ON, et al. Geographical Prevalence of Polycystic Ovary Syndrome as Determined by Region and Race/Ethnicity. Int J Environ Res Public Health 2018;15(11):2589.
3. He Y, Lu Y, Zhu Q, et al. Influence of metabolic syndrome on female fertility and in vitro fertilization outcomes in PCOS women. Am J Obstet Gynecol 2019;221(2): 138.e1-12.
4. Balen AH, Morley LC, Misso M, et al. The management of anovulatory infertility in women with polycystic ovary syndrome: an analysis of the evidence to support the development of global WHO guidance. Hum Reprod Update 2016;22(6):687–708.
5. Sha T, Wang X, Cheng W, et al. A meta-analysis of pregnancy-related outcomes and complications in women with polycystic ovary syndrome undergoing IVF. Reprod Biomed Online 2019;39(2):281–93.
6. Roos N, Kieler H, Sahlin L, et al. Risk of adverse pregnancy outcomes in women with polycystic ovary syndrome: population based cohort study. BMJ 2011;343: d6309.
7. Yu HF, Chen HS, Rao DP, et al. Association between polycystic ovary syndrome and the risk of pregnancy complications: A PRISMA-compliant systematic review and meta-analysis. Medicine (Baltimore) 2016;95(51):e4863.
8. Palomba S, de Wilde MA, Falbo A, et al. Pregnancy complications in women with polycystic ovary syndrome. Hum Reprod Update 2015;21(5):575–92.
9. Goodman NF, Cobin RH, Futterweit W, et al. American Association of Clinical Endocrinologists, American College of Endocrinology, and androgen excess and PCOS society disease state clinical review: guide to the best practices in the evaluation and treatment of polycystic ovary syndrome - part 2. Endocr Pract 2015;21(12):1415–26.

10. Teede HJ, Misso ML, Costello MF, et al. Recommendations from the international evidence-based guideline for the assessment and management of polycystic ovary syndrome. Hum Reprod 2018;33(9):1602–18.
11. ACOG Practice Bulletin No. 190: Gestational Diabetes Mellitus. Obstet Gynecol 2018;131(2):e49–64.
12. ACOG Practice Bulletin No. 202: Gestational Hypertension and Preeclampsia. Obstet Gynecol 2019;133(1):e1–25.
13. Palomba S, Falbo A, Russo T, et al. Pregnancy in women with polycystic ovary syndrome: the effect of different phenotypes and features on obstetric and neonatal outcomes. Fertil Steril 2010;94(5):1805–11.
14. Mumm H, Jensen DM, Sørensen JA, et al. Hyperandrogenism and phenotypes of polycystic ovary syndrome are not associated with differences in obstetric outcomes. Acta Obstet Gynecol Scand 2015;94(2):204–11.
15. Boomsma CM, Eijkemans MJ, Hughes EG, et al. A meta-analysis of pregnancy outcomes in women with polycystic ovary syndrome. Hum Reprod Update 2006;12(6):673–83.
16. Qin JZ, Pang LH, Li MJ, et al. Obstetric complications in women with polycystic ovary syndrome: a systematic review and meta-analysis. Reprod Biol Endocrinol 2013;11:56.
17. de Wilde MA, Veltman-Verhulst SM, Goverde AJ, et al. Preconception predictors of gestational diabetes: a multicentre prospective cohort study on the predominant complication of pregnancy in polycystic ovary syndrome. Hum Reprod 2014;29(6):1327–36.
18. Köninger A, Iannaccone A, Hajder E, et al. Afamin predicts gestational diabetes in polycystic ovary syndrome patients preconceptionally. Endocr Connect 2019; 8(5):616–24.
19. Zheng W, Huang W, Zhang L, et al. Early pregnancy metabolic factors associated with gestational diabetes mellitus in normal-weight women with polycystic ovary syndrome: a two-phase cohort study. Diabetol Metab Syndr 2019;11:71.
20. Dutton H, Borengasser SJ, Gaudet LM, et al. Obesity in Pregnancy: Optimizing Outcomes for Mom and Baby. Med Clin North Am 2018;102(1):87–106.
21. Brosens I, Pijnenborg R, Vercruysse L, et al. The "Great Obstetrical Syndromes" are associated with disorders of deep placentation. Am J Obstet Gynecol 2011; 204(3):193–201.
22. Koster MP, de Wilde MA, Veltman-Verhulst SM, et al. Placental characteristics in women with polycystic ovary syndrome. Hum Reprod 2015;30(12):2829–37.
23. Kuo K, Roberts VHJ, Gaffney J, et al. Maternal High-Fat Diet Consumption and Chronic Hyperandrogenemia Are Associated With Placental Dysfunction in Female Rhesus Macaques. Endocrinology 2019;160(8):1937–49.
24. Kelley AS, Smith YR, Padmanabhan V. A Narrative Review of Placental Contribution to Adverse Pregnancy Outcomes in Women With Polycystic Ovary Syndrome. J Clin Endocrinol Metab 2019;104(11):5299–315.
25. Barker DJ, Thornburg KL. The obstetric origins of health for a lifetime. Clin Obstet Gynecol 2013;56(3):511–9.
26. Vanky E, Engen Hanem LG, Abbott DH. Children born to women with polycystic ovary syndrome-short- and long-term impacts on health and development. Fertil Steril 2019;111(6):1065–75.
27. Doherty DA, Newnham JP, Bower C, et al. Implications of polycystic ovary syndrome for pregnancy and for the health of offspring. Obstet Gynecol 2015; 125(6):1397–406.

28. Gu L, Liu H, Gu X, et al. Metabolic control of oocyte development: linking maternal nutrition and reproductive outcomes. Cell Mol Life Sci 2015;72(2):251–71.
29. Forsum E, Brantsæter AL, Olafsdottir AS, et al. Weight loss before conception: A systematic literature review. Food Nutr Res 2013;57.
30. Schummers L, Hutcheon JA, Bodnar LM, et al. Risk of adverse pregnancy outcomes by prepregnancy body mass index: a population-based study to inform prepregnancy weight loss counseling. Obstet Gynecol 2015;125(1):133–43.
31. Lim SS, Hutchison SK, Van Ryswyk E, et al. Lifestyle changes in women with polycystic ovary syndrome. Cochrane Database Syst Rev 2019;(3):CD007506.
32. Legro RS, Dodson WC, Kunselman AR, et al. Benefit of Delayed Fertility Therapy With Preconception Weight Loss Over Immediate Therapy in Obese Women With PCOS. J Clin Endocrinol Metab 2016;101(7):2658–66.
33. Yanovski SZ, Yanovski JA. Long-term drug treatment for obesity: a systematic and clinical review. JAMA 2014;311(1):74–86.
34. Falcone V, Stopp T, Feichtinger M, et al. Pregnancy after bariatric surgery: a narrative literature review and discussion of impact on pregnancy management and outcome. BMC Pregnancy Childbirth 2018;18(1):507.
35. Dokras A, Stener-Victorin E, Yildiz BO, et al. Androgen Excess- Polycystic Ovary Syndrome Society: position statement on depression, anxiety, quality of life, and eating disorders in polycystic ovary syndrome. Fertil Steril 2018;109(5):888–99.
36. Brutocao C, Zaiem F, Alsawas M, et al. Psychiatric disorders in women with polycystic ovary syndrome: a systematic review and meta-analysis. Endocrine 2018; 62(2):318–25.
37. O'Connor E, Senger CA, Henninger ML, et al. Interventions to Prevent Perinatal Depression: Evidence Report and Systematic Review for the US Preventive Services Task Force. JAMA 2019;321(6):588–601.
38. Andersen M, Glintborg D. Diagnosis and follow-up of type 2 diabetes in women with PCOS: a role for OGTT? Eur J Endocrinol 2018;179(3):D1–14.
39. 2. Classification and Diagnosis of Diabetes: Standards of Medical Care in Diabetes-2020. Diabetes Care 2020;43(Suppl 1):S14–31.
40. Dominguez JE, Street L, Louis J. Management of Obstructive Sleep Apnea in Pregnancy. Obstet Gynecol Clin North Am 2018;45(2):233–47.
41. Farabi SS, Barbour LA, Heiss K, et al. Obstructive Sleep Apnea is Associated with Altered Glycemic Patterns in Pregnant Women with Obesity. J Clin Endocrinol Metab 2019;104(7):2569–79.
42. Kahal H, Kyrou I, Tahrani AA, et al. Obstructive sleep apnoea and polycystic ovary syndrome: A comprehensive review of clinical interactions and underlying pathophysiology. Clin Endocrinol (Oxf) 2017;87(4):313–9.
43. Barbour LA, Scifres C, Valent AM, et al. A Cautionary Response to SMFM Statement: Pharmacological Treatment of Gestational Diabetes. Am J Obstet Gynecol 2018;219(4):367.e1-7.
44. Barbour LA, Feig DS. Metformin for Gestational Diabetes Mellitus: Progeny, Perspective, and a Personalized Approach. Diabetes Care 2019;42(3):396–9.
45. Bidhendi Yarandi R, Behboudi-Gandevani S, Amiri M, et al. Metformin therapy before conception versus throughout the pregnancy and risk of gestational diabetes mellitus in women with polycystic ovary syndrome: a systemic review, meta-analysis and meta-regression. Diabetol Metab Syndr 2019;11:58.
46. Doi SAR, Furuya-Kanamori L, Toft E, et al. Metformin in pregnancy to avert gestational diabetes in women at high risk: Meta-analysis of randomized controlled trials. Obes Rev 2020;21(1):e12964.

47. Tan X, Li S, Chang Y, et al. Effect of metformin treatment during pregnancy on women with PCOS: a systematic review and meta-analysis. Clin Invest Med 2016;39(4):E120–31.

48. Role of metformin for ovulation induction in infertile patients with polycystic ovary syndrome (PCOS): a guideline. Fertil Steril 2017;108(3):426–41.

49. Vanky E, Stridsklev S, Heimstad R, et al. Metformin versus placebo from first trimester to delivery in polycystic ovary syndrome: a randomized, controlled multicenter study. J Clin Endocrinol Metab 2010;95(12):E448–55.

50. Løvvik TS, Carlsen SM, Salvesen Ø, et al. Use of metformin to treat pregnant women with polycystic ovary syndrome (PregMet2): a randomised, double-blind, placebo-controlled trial. Lancet Diabetes Endocrinol 2019;7(4):256–66.

51. Feng L, Lin XF, Wan ZH, et al. Efficacy of metformin on pregnancy complications in women with polycystic ovary syndrome: a meta-analysis. Gynecol Endocrinol 2015;31(11):833–9.

52. Dodd JM, Grivell RM, Deussen AR, et al. Metformin for women who are over-weight or obese during pregnancy for improving maternal and infant outcomes. Cochrane Database Syst Rev 2018;(7):CD010564.

53. Romero R, Erez O, Hüttemann M, et al. Metformin, the aspirin of the 21st century: its role in gestational diabetes mellitus, prevention of preeclampsia and cancer, and the promotion of longevity. Am J Obstet Gynecol 2017;217(3):282–302.

54. Kalafat E, Sukur YE, Abdi A, et al. Metformin for prevention of hypertensive dis-orders of pregnancy in women with gestational diabetes or obesity: systematic review and meta-analysis of randomized trials. Ultrasound Obstet Gynecol 2018;52(6):706–14.

55. Underdal MO, Stridsklev S, Oppen IH, et al. Does Metformin Treatment During Pregnancy Modify the Future Metabolic Profile in Women With PCOS? J Clin Endocrinol Metab 2018;103(6):2408–13.

56. Aroda VR, Christophi CA, Edelstein SL, et al. The effect of lifestyle intervention and metformin on preventing or delaying diabetes among women with and without gestational diabetes: the Diabetes Prevention Program outcomes study 10-year follow-up. J Clin Endocrinol Metab 2015;100(4):1646–53.

57. Ratner RE, Christophi CA, Metzger BE, et al. Prevention of diabetes in women with a history of gestational diabetes: effects of metformin and lifestyle interventions. J Clin Endocrinol Metab 2008;93(12):4774–9.

58. Gonzalez CD, Alvariñas J, Bagnes MFG, et al. Metformin and Pregnancy Out-comes: Evidence Gaps and Unanswered Questions. Curr Clin Pharmacol 2019;14(1):54–60.

59. Priya G, Kalra S. Metformin in the management of diabetes during pregnancy and lactation. Drugs Context 2018;7:212523.

60. Lindsay RS, Loeken MR. Metformin use in pregnancy: promises and uncer-tainties. Diabetologia 2017;60(9):1612–9.

61. Carlsen SM, Martinussen MP, Vanky E. Metformin's effect on first-year weight gain: a follow-up study. Pediatrics 2012;130(5):e1222–6.

62. Ro TB, Ludvigsen HV, Carlsen SM, et al. Growth, body composition and meta-bolic profile of 8-year-old children exposed to metformin in utero. Scand J Clin Lab Invest 2012;72(7):570–5.

63. Hanem LGE, Stridsklev S, Juliusson PB, et al. Metformin Use in PCOS Pregnan-cies Increases the Risk of Offspring Overweight at 4 Years of Age: Follow-Up of Two RCTs. J Clin Endocrinol Metab 2018;103(4):1612–21.

64. Hanem LGE, Salvesen Ø, Juliusson PB, et al. Intrauterine metformin exposure and offspring cardiometabolic risk factors (PedMet study): a 5-10 year follow-up of the

PregMet randomised controlled trial. Lancet Child Adolesc Health 2019;3(3): 166–74.

65. Greger HK, Hanem LGE, Østgård HF, et al. Cognitive function in metformin exposed children, born to mothers with PCOS - follow-up of an RCT. BMC Pediatr 2020;20(1):60.

66. Rowan JA, Hague WM, Gao W, et al. Metformin versus insulin for the treatment of gestational diabetes. N Engl J Med 2008;358(19):2003–15.

67. Tarry-Adkins JL, Aiken CE, Ozanne SE. Neonatal, infant, and childhood growth following metformin versus insulin treatment for gestational diabetes: A systematic review and meta-analysis. Plos Med 2019;16(8):e1002848.

68. van Weelden W, Wekker V, de Wit L, et al. Long-Term Effects of Oral Antidiabetic Drugs During Pregnancy on Offspring: A Systematic Review and Meta-analysis of Follow-up Studies of RCTs. Diabetes Ther 2018;9(5):1811–29.

69. Feig DS, Donovan LE, Zinman B, et al. Metformin in women with type 2 diabetes in pregnancy (MiTy): a multicentre, international, randomised, placebo-controlled trial. Lancet Diabetes Endocrinol 2020;8(10):834–44.

70. Panagiotopoulou O, Syngelaki A, Georgiopoulos G, et al. Metformin use in obese mothers is associated with improved cardiovascular profile in the offspring. Am J Obstet Gynecol 2020;223(2):246.e1-10.

71. ACOG Committee Opinion No. 736: Optimizing Postpartum Care. Obstet Gynecol 2018;131(5):e140–50.

72. ACOG Committee Opinion No. 757: Screening for Perinatal Depression. Obstet Gynecol 2018;132(5):e208–12.

73. March WA, Whitrow MJ, Davies MJ, et al. Postnatal depression in a community-based study of women with polycystic ovary syndrome. Acta Obstet Gynecol Scand 2018;97(7):838–44.

74. Harrison CL, Teede HJ, Joham AE, et al. Breastfeeding and obesity in PCOS. Expert Rev Endocrinol Metab 2016;11(6):449–54.

75. Joham AE, Nanayakkara N, Ranasinha S, et al. Obesity, polycystic ovary syndrome and breastfeeding: an observational study. Acta Obstet Gynecol Scand 2016;95(4):458–66.

76. Gunderson EP, Hurston SR, Ning X, et al. Lactation and Progression to Type 2 Diabetes Mellitus After Gestational Diabetes Mellitus: A Prospective Cohort Study. Ann Intern Med 2015;163(12):889–98.

77. Crume TL, Ogden L, Daniels S, et al. The impact of in utero exposure to diabetes on childhood body mass index growth trajectories: the EPOCH study. J Pediatr 2011;158(6):941–6.

78. Nicklas JM, Barbour LA. Optimizing Weight for Maternal and Infant Health - Tenable, or Too Late? Expert Rev Endocrinol Metab 2015;10(2):227–42.

79. Aroda VR, Knowler WC, Crandall JP, et al. Metformin for diabetes prevention: insights gained from the Diabetes Prevention Program/Diabetes Prevention Program Outcomes Study. Diabetologia 2017;60(9):1601–11.

80. Herman WH. The cost-effectiveness of diabetes prevention: results from the Diabetes Prevention Program and the Diabetes Prevention Program Outcomes Study. Clin Diabetes Endocrinol 2015;1:9.

81. Briggs GG, Ambrose PJ, Nageotte MP, et al. Excretion of metformin into breast milk and the effect on nursing infants. Obstet Gynecol 2005;105(6):1437–41.

Genetics of Polycystic Ovary Syndrome: What is New?

Corrine K. Welt, MD

KEYWORDS

- Genetics • Precision medicine • Mendelian randomization

KEY POINTS

- Using available genetic data, the current polygenic risk scores do not reach sufficient diagnostic ability for clinical use.
- Subtypes of polycystic ovary syndrome (PCOS) may be identified through analysis of genetic risk variants.
- Precision medicine for PCOS requires larger studies and the ability to integrate many variables into diagnostic decision-making and treatment.

GENETIC VARIANTS CONFER RISK FOR POLYCYSTIC OVARY SYNDROME

Polycystic ovary syndrome (PCOS) remains the most common endocrinopathy in reproductive age women, with lifetime costs for diagnosis and treatment estimated in the billions of dollars.[1] The cause has been difficult to identify despite years of physiologic studies. Further, the diagnosis in adolescents may be masked by normal developmental changes.[2] Thus, early intervention and prevention strategies are not available. In adults, the broad diagnostic criteria encompass a heterogeneous patient population. Although some patients have increased risk for type 2 diabetes and metabolic consequences, others seem to suffer mainly from infertility related to irregular menses.[3–5] Therefore, future health implications are difficult to predict in an individual patient.

Genetic variants could provide the critical predictive risk information for the development of PCOS and PCOS comorbidities. PCOS is highly heritable.[6] The tetrachoric correlation for PCOS, a correlation used for binary data, is twice as high in monozygotic twins (0.71 [0.43–0.88]) compared with dizygotic twins (0.38 [0.00–0.66]), suggesting PCOS is approximately 79% influenced by genetic variance.[6] Although twin studies are the strongest to estimate genetic risk, many additional studies have demonstrated familial clustering of PCOS, with approximately 50% of sisters sharing PCOS features.[7] Although this pattern of inheritance in sisters suggested a dominant

Division of Endocrinology, Metabolism and Diabetes, University of Utah School of Medicine, 15 North 2030 East, 2110A, Salt Lake City, UT 84112, USA
E-mail address: cwelt@genetics.utah.edu

Endocrinol Metab Clin N Am 50 (2021) 71–82
https://doi.org/10.1016/j.ecl.2020.10.006
0889-8529/21/© 2020 Elsevier Inc. All rights reserved.

endo.theclinics.com

mode of inheritance, it is now clear that PCOS is a complex, polygenic disorder in which multiple risk loci with small effects contribute to disease, similar to the genetics of type 2 diabetes.[8–10]

Great leaps in genetics came with the mapping of the human genome, the realization that most of the DNA variation is shared at high rates across all humans, and the understanding that multiple DNA variants are inherited together in blocks (linkage disequilibrium [LD]). Scientists used the new knowledge to develop genotype arrays, with representative DNA variants found in 1% or more of the population, covering a significant portion of the LD blocks across the human genome.[11,12] Genome-wide association studies (GWAS) used these arrays to identify risk variants that were overrepresented in disease cases compared with controls. Because the number of DNA variants tested was so large, approaching one million, the P value indicating a significant association must be very low ($<5 \times 10^{-8}$).[12] In addition, the effect sizes of these common variants are small, requiring tens to hundreds of thousands of participants to demonstrate effects. Thus, the use of these approaches to understand PCOS has been a challenge.

The initial GWASs were performed in Han Chinese subjects, demonstrating 11 gene loci associated with PCOS (**Table 1**).[9,10] Our group and others found that several of these loci also confer risk for PCOS in European women.[13–19] Additional loci emerged from meta-analyses and replication in large groups of European women.[17,18] These studies culminated in the largest PCOS GWAS from the International PCOS Consortium, which included a meta-analysis of 10,074 PCOS cases and 103,164 controls.[20] Together, there were a total of 19 loci that confer risk for PCOS in Han Chinese and European women (see **Table 1**).

The next wave of GWAS will capitalize on large DNA collections agnostic to disease and linked to electronic medical records to identify cases and controls using International Classification of Disease (ICD) codes or more complicated algorithms. Using the Partners Healthcare electronic medical records, ICD codes performed equivalently to an algorithm validated to identify PCOS cases using natural language processing.[21] Supporting the use of ICD codes for PCOS identification, the first GWAS using electronic medical records to pull PCOS cases replicated 2 previously identified loci from the International PCOS consortium and located 2 additional loci (see **Table 1**).[22] The study also identified the first locus in African American women.[22] The stage is now set for further studies using larger numbers and expanding the ethnicities examined.

IS GENETIC ARCHITECTURE THE SAME FOR ALL POLYCYSTIC OVARY SYNDROME SUBTYPES?

A robust discussion always ensues when the criteria for PCOS are discussed (see Sydney Chang and Andrea Dunaif's article, "Diagnosis of Polycystic Ovary Syndrome: Which Criteria to Use When?," in this issue). Although there was concern that using National Institutes of Health (NIH), Rotterdam and self-reported PCOS would dilute the ability to identify genetic risk for PCOS, the problem did not materialize. In fact, the genetic architecture was similar across the diagnostic subtypes, with the exception of one locus, *GATA4/NEIL2,* which demonstrated heterogeneity of effect.[20] At this locus, the most significant association was demonstrated in subjects defined using the NIH criteria (odds ratio for risk [OR] 1.33; 1.26–1.41 95% confidence interval) and the lowest for self-report (OR 1.08; 1.03–1.13), although all were risk loci. Taken together with validation of PCOS cases from the electronic record, large studies using electronic datasets to isolate all subtypes of PCOS will be valid.

Table 1
Single nucleotide polymorphisms associated with polycystic ovary syndrome at genome-wide significance

	Chromosome:Position	Risk Variant/ Reference Variant	Nearest Gene	Associated Phenotypes[a]	References
Han Chinese Only	2:48978159	A/G	LHCGR		9
	12:66224461	A/C	HMGA2		10
	19:7166109	A/G	INSR		10
	20:52447303	A/G	SUMO1P1		10
Both	2:43721508	T/C	THADA	PCOM, Increased T	9,20,36
	2:43561780	A/G			
	2:49247832	T/C	FSHR	Increased FSH, OD	9,20
	2:213391766	A/G	ERRB4	OD, PCOM	20,22,52
	2:212291772	A/G			
	9:97648587	A/G	C9orf3	HA, OD, PCOM	9,20
	9:97723266	A/G			
	9:126525212	A/G	DENND1A	HA, OD, PCOM	9,20,22
	9:126619233	A/G			
	11:30226356	T/C	ARL14EP/FSHB	Decreased FSH, Increased LH, OD	20,53
	11:102070639	A/G	YAP1	OD, PCOM	10,20
	11:102043240	A/G			
	12:56390636	A/G	ERBB3/RAB5	HA, OD, PCOM	10,20
	12:56477694	T/A			
	16:52347819	T/G	TOX3	HA	10,20
	16:52375777				

(continued on next page)

Table 1
(continued)

Chromosome:Position	Risk Variant/ Reference Variant	Nearest Gene	Associated Phenotypes[a]	References
European				
3:149319873	C/T	*WWTR1*	OD	22
5:131813204	T/C	*IRF1/RAD50*	Increased testosterone	20
6:159898261	C/T	*SOD2*	HA, PCOM	22
8:11623889	A/T	*GATA4INEIL2*	OD, PCOM	20
9:5440589	A/C	*PLGRKT*		20
11:113949232	T/C	*ZBTB16*	OD, PCOM	20
12:75941042	C/T	*KRR1*	OD	20
20:31420757	T/A	*MAPRE1*		20

[a] HA, hyperandrogenism; OD, ovulatory dysfunction; PCOM, polycystic ovary morphology.
Data from Refs.[9,10,20,22,36,52,53]

In addition to studying larger datasets, it is time to determine what the risk means and how to move our expanding scientific understanding to clinically applicable diagnostic and treatment options.

MOVING FROM GENOTYPE TO FUNCTIONAL MECHANISM—HOW DOES A RISK VARIANT CAUSE POLYCYSTIC OVARY SYNDROME?

Identifying the underlying function of the GWAS risk variants has been difficult because most of them are noncoding and reside in introns and between genes where a mechanism is not apparent. It has also been estimated that only one-third of the associated variants affect the nearest gene.[12] Nevertheless, approximately 60% of the common variants associated with disease map to regions of DNA hypersensitivity and regulatory regions.[23,24] Investigators have capitalized on these properties in other diseases to determine the mechanism through which variants associated with low-density lipoprotein cholesterol levels, autoimmune disorders, and Crohn disease cause risk.[23,25,26] Elucidating the underlying mechanism that ties a common variant to disease risk requires examining regulatory influence and the associated gene expression.

The risk variants identified near *FSHβ* (rs11031006 and s11031005) illustrate a regulatory mechanism for genome-wide associated variants. The rs11031006 and rs11031005 variants not only confer risk for PCOS but are also associated with lower FSH and higher luteinizing hormone (LH) levels.[17,18,27,28] The association between rs11031006 and PCOS risk disappears when the relationship is controlled for LH levels, suggesting that PCOS risk at the FSH locus is driven by gonadotropin dysregulation.[18] The rs11031006 and s11031005 risk variants are located 26 kilobases proximal to the FSHβ promoter.[17,18,27] The region of interest is located approximately 500 bases downstream from a histone H3 mono-methylation of the fourth lysine residue (H3K4Me1) enhancer site and 2000 bases upstream from open chromatin sites (identified by DNase-Seq). H3K4Me1 and histone H3 acetylation of the 27th lysine residue (H3K27Ac) enhancer sites were identified at rs11031006 in a lymphoblastoid cell line, along with a H3K4me1 enhancer site in 2 stem cell lines and induced pluripotent stem cells, pointing to the role of the region in gene regulation.[29,30] Co-accessibility analysis demonstrated an open, putative cis-regulatory region at the site, and disruption of the conserved locus in a mouse gonadotrope cell line resulted in increased *Fshb* expression and FSH protein secretion.[31] Expression of an additional candidate gene located within the same LD block, ADP ribosylation factor such as GTPase 14 effector protein (ARL14EP), did not change.[31–33] Taken together, the human DNA features, co-accessibility study, and mouse experimental cell line data provide evidence that this risk locus affects a regulatory region for *FSHβ*. The additional effect of the risk variants on LH levels may be the result of decreased estradiol or the relative excess of *Cga*, because in mice with *Fshb* deleted, *Lhb* expression and LH secretion is increased.[34,35] Ongoing research will determine how the region regulates FSH secretion, focusing on the stimulatory hormones involved, transcription factors affected, and three-dimensional interactions with the FSH promoter.[31]

There is growing evidence that some of the genetic variants play a role in PCOS risk through testosterone regulation. The *IRF1/RAD50* locus was the only locus associated with testosterone levels in the European GWAS.[20] However, the association was not found in a GWAS of testosterone levels[36] and may therefore play a role through indirect effects on testosterone or follicle number. Instead, the GWAS of testosterone levels found *THADA* and *FSHβ* loci are important testosterone regulators in women.[36] The relationship between the *FSHβ* locus and testosterone may occur through the elevated LH levels, whereas the *THADA* PCOS risk locus is found approximately 150 bp from a H3K27Ac enhancer site and may, therefore, also mark a regulatory site.[30]

Other work has examined the genetic locus containing *DENND1A,* a risk locus that has been replicated in Han Chinese and European women.[9,20,22] The gene variant within the intron of *DENND1A* is associated with hyperandrogenism, defined using both clinical and biochemical criteria.[19,20] When DENND1A.v2 splice variant found at increased levels in theca cells from women with PCOS was overexpressed in a theca cell line, androgen biosynthesis and *CYP17A1*expression increased, whereas knockdown of the transcript in PCOS theca cells reduced androgen production and *CYP17A1* mRNA.[37] However, the heterozygote in a mouse model in which *DENND1A* was deleted had no fertility or adult phenotype.[38] The homozygous deletion was embryonic lethal but did result in abnormal brain development and a decrease in primordial germ cell number and differentiation in the fetus.[38] In another mouse model expressing human *DENND1A.v2* mRNA, protein was not measurable, but *CYP17A1* mRNA expression increased, as did androstenedione secretion from ex vivo theca cells.[39] However, *DENND1A* variants have not been associated with testosterone levels, per se, in any study. Taken together, the variants in the intron of *DENND1A* affect the degree of hyperandrogenism, but it remains to be determined whether the PCOS variants are acting through *DENND1A* mRNA levels or whether the variant might have a role in regulating another nearby gene.

MENDELIAN RANDOMIZATION—WHAT DOES IT TELL US?

Mendelian randomization is a statistical approach used in genetic studies to determine whether an exposure, measured by a genetically influenced trait such as obesity, has a causal effect on a disease of interest (PCOS).[40] The approach quantifies whether the genetic risk for the exposure influences the presence of the disease. The approach assumes that the trait or exposure (obesity) has a completely independent genetic architecture from PCOS and that any genetic risk for obesity should be randomly distributed in genomes from women with PCOS because the risk genes are not linked, that is, located very close in proximity on the chromosomes. In a simplified manner, any obesity gene risk variant would be found at equal frequency in PCOS cases and controls if there was no causal relationship between obesity and PCOS.

Using the Mendelian randomization approach, genetic determinants for traits including body mass index (BMI), fasting insulin, depression, male pattern balding, and age at menopause are found at increased frequency in PCOS.[20] These traits are therefore considered causal for PCOS, reinforcing previous observational studies. The male pattern balding thus presents itself as a male phenotype for PCOS, as has been hypothesized in the past.[41]

Mendelian randomization has been approached in the reverse fashion, examining whether PCOS causes obesity. In the reverse sense, the exposure is taken as PCOS and the outcome obesity.[42] However, the PCOS exposure is based on the relatively small GWAS, to date. More accurately, one could look at testosterone levels, which are heritable and a critical component of PCOS.[36] A large Mendelian randomization study of genetic variants determining testosterone levels confirmed the causal relationship between higher testosterone and PCOS.[36] The study also demonstrated a causal relationship between bioavailable testosterone and type 2 diabetes in women, likely driven by SHBG levels, which are known to be inversely related to insulin resistance.[36] In men, genetic determinants of testosterone were associated with decreased type 2 diabetes risk in the same study. These data point to the possibility that PCOS risk through intrinsic increases in testosterone may not have the same metabolic risk in men in the same families.

GENETIC RISK SCORES—ARE THEY CLINICALLY USEFUL FOR POLYCYSTIC OVARY SYNDROME DIAGNOSIS?

Ideally, clinicians need a test that will predict risk of PCOS before the onset of symptoms, so that they can intervene early. Polygenic (genetic) risk scores for PCOS could provide the needed predictive information. A polygenic risk score is a construct of the probability of disease posed by common genetic risk variants, with each variant weighted based on the relative influence of the variant on the disease. The area under the curve of the receiver operator characteristic (ROC) measures the discriminatory power of a polygenic risk score to detect disease. The closer the area under the ROC curve to 1, the better the disease discrimination. As an example, the predictive value of the polygenic risk score for coronary artery disease using common genetic variants is 0.79 to 0.8 and identifies 8% of the population at 3-fold risk for coronary artery disease.[43] The polygenic risk score of common variants identifies up to 20 times greater numbers than familial hypercholesterolemia rare variants for coronary artery disease and outperformed risk detection from clinical risk assessment (family history, cholesterol levels hypertension).[43] Although a genetic risk score can be used at any age, one could add historical or phenotypic risk factors such as BMI to improve its predictive ability.

These models depend on the availability of large GWAS studies, ensuring that the known genetic risk variants capture a sufficient proportion of the genetic risk for PCOS. Unfortunately to date, PCOS GWASs have not reached these threshold levels in women of European and Han Chinese ancestry and have not begun to examine genetic risk in other ethnic populations to any significant degree. A genetic risk score using the most up-to-date GWAS resulted in an area under the ROC curve of 0.54 to 0.72 for detecting PCOS in women of European ancestry.[20,44] The best model did not perform as well in women of African American ancestry with the ROC area under the curve only 0.54.[44] Therefore, the discriminatory value of these calculated genetic risk scores are not yet clinically useful.

Understanding the discriminatory limitations in PCOS, the polygenic risk score was used in a phenome-wide association study to identify comorbid PCOS disease from electronic medical records using ICD codes.[44] The phenotypes are hypothesized to be associated with PCOS risk, as they are identified using the polygenic risk score marking predisposition for PCOS. When the polygenic risk score was used to identify associated phenotypes across an electronic dataset of more than 120,000 subjects, the score was associated with polycystic ovaries, as expected. The score was also associated with morbid obesity and type 2 diabetes in men and women, along with hypercholesterolemia, disorders of lipid metabolism, hypertension, and sleep apnea in women.[44] In a second phenome-wide study, an association was found between 3 individual genome-wide significant risk variants and mental health disorders, providing support for the previous Mendelian Randomization studies.[22]

Even with future development of an accurate polygenic risk score for PCOS, it is not clear that a predictive test will be sufficient to change behavior of patients and physicians to prevent disease. For example, obesity is a causal factor for PCOS risk.[20] Nevertheless, previous studies examining the possibility that genetic risk will change behavior determined that behavior was not changed by predicted risk.[45]

PRECISION MEDICINE FOR POLYCYSTIC OVARY SYNDROME

Precision medicine integrates genetic, environment, and lifestyle risks to stratify patients and provide individualized diagnosis and treatment plans. These individualized diagnosis and treatment plans are targeted to the underlying cause of the disease and should improve patient outcome. Ideally, precision medicine will break PCOS down into tractable subsets based on disease risk. Although no striking subphenotypes emerged when examining the components of the PCOS diagnosis,[20] risk categories are beginning to stand out. The *FSHβ* locus points to a gonadotropin cause.[18,20] The *DENND1A*, *THADA*, and *IRF1/RAD50* loci are associated with hyperandrogenism or testosterone levels.[20,36] The *ERBB4*, *YAP1*, and *ZBTB16* loci are associated with ovulatory dysfunction and polycystic ovary morphology, perhaps alluding to a role in follicular function and fertility.[20] Although the polygenic risk score measures the contribution of genetic risk from all potential pathways combined, it is possible that splitting risk up into individually contributing pathways may help target treatment and symptoms. Larger studies are needed to perform such an analysis.

Clinically, precision medicine should improve treatment. When we examined the LH and FSH response to GnRH stimulation (n = 14), women with PCOS who carried the *FSHβ* rs11031006 risk allele had increased mean LH levels (28.3 ± 0.04 vs 22.1 ± 5.5 IU/L; $P<.05$) and an increased GnRH-stimulated LH response (LH area under the curve 19,624 ± 2336 vs 7362 ± 2179 IU/L min^{-1}; $P<.05$).[46] In addition, carriers of the rs11031006 risk variant demonstrated a decreased ovulatory response to clomiphene citrate ($X^2 = 7.3$; $P = .007$).[47] Together, these data point to an altered gonadotropin response to GnRH stimulation and estrogen receptor blockade that may be detrimental for fertility treatment in women with PCOS who already have high LH levels. Developing specific treatments to precisely manipulate the *FSHβ* locus could target therapy to increase FSH and decrease LH secretion.

Two lines of evidence point to obesity as a critical causal factor for PCOS. The Mendelian randomization studies demonstrate obesity as a causal factor.[20] The phenome-wide association study demonstrates it as a comorbid association.[22] Obesity also worsens the hyperandrogenism and menstrual irregularity.[4,48] Therefore, targeting obesity in those at particular genetic or environmental risk could prevent the full PCOS phenotype or prevent disease altogether.

Implementing precision medicine to diagnose and treat PCOS depends on several factors. First, we need to capture a greater component of genetic variation in GWAS. The size of the current PCOS GWAS cohorts are relatively small compared with GWASs that have been performed for CAD and type 2 diabetes.[20,43,49] PCOS GWAS are also limited in ethnic diversity and depth.[49] We will need to incorporate lifestyle factors such as weight and weight trajectory, which can influence the clinical manifestations of PCOS.[44,50] We also need to determine whether environmental factors play a role, as has been suggested by exposures to endocrine-disrupting chemicals and changes in the individual's microbiome.[51] A comprehensive look will need to capture electronic health data, genomics, proteomics, metabolomics, environmental exposures, and tracked or self-reported data.

CLINICS CARE POINTS

- Polycystic ovary syndrome has a complex genetic architecture.

- Polygenic risk scores are not yet sufficiently robust for clinical use.
- Polycystic ovary syndrome subtypes may be defined in the future through personalized genetic risk.

DISCLOSURE

Eunice Kennedy Shriver National Institute of Child Health and Human Development (R01HD065029); American Diabetes Association (1_10_CT-57).

REFERENCES

1. Azziz R, Marin C, Hoq L, et al. Health care-related economic burden of the polycystic ovary syndrome during the reproductive life span. J Clin Endocrinol Metab 2005;90(8):4650–8.
2. Legro RS, Arslanian SA, Ehrmann DA, et al. Diagnosis and treatment of polycystic ovary syndrome: an endocrine society clinical practice guideline. J Clin Endocrinol Metab 2013;98(12):4565–92.
3. Dewailly D, Catteau-Jonard S, Reyss AC, et al. Oligoanovulation with polycystic ovaries but not overt hyperandrogenism. J Clin Endocrinol Metab 2006;91(10): 3922–7.
4. Welt CK, Gudmundsson JA, Arason G, et al. Characterizing discrete subsets of polycystic ovary syndrome as defined by the Rotterdam criteria: the impact of weight on phenotype and metabolic features. J Clin Endocrinol Metab 2006; 91(12):4842–8.
5. Barber TM, Wass JA, McCarthy MI, et al. Metabolic characteristics of women with polycystic ovaries and oligo-amenorrhoea but normal androgen levels: implications for the management of polycystic ovary syndrome. Clin Endocrinol 2007; 66(4):513–7.
6. Vink JM, Sadrzadeh S, Lambalk CB, et al. Heritability of polycystic ovary syndrome in a Dutch twin-family study. J Clin Endocrinol Metab 2006;91(6):2100–4.
7. Legro RS, Driscoll D, Strauss JF 3rd, et al. Evidence for a genetic basis for hyperandrogenemia in polycystic ovary syndrome. Proc Natl Acad Sci U S A 1998; 95(25):14956–60.
8. Florez JC. Genetic susceptibility for polycystic ovary syndrome on chromosome 19: advances in the genetic dissection of complex reproductive traits. J Clin Endocrinol Metab 2005;90(12):6732–4.
9. Chen ZJ, Zhao H, He L, et al. Genome-wide association study identifies susceptibility loci for polycystic ovary syndrome on chromosome 2p16.3, 2p21 and 9q33.3. Nat Genet 2011;43(1):55–9.
10. Shi Y, Zhao H, Shi Y, et al. Genome-wide association study identifies eight new risk loci for polycystic ovary syndrome. Nat Genet 2012;44(9):1020–5.
11. International HapMap C. The international hapmap project. Nature 2003; 426(6968):789–96.
12. Visscher PM, Wray NR, Zhang Q, et al. 10 Years of GWAS discovery: biology, function, and translation. Am J Hum Genet 2017;101(1):5–22.
13. Welt CK, Styrkarsdottir U, Ehrmann DA, et al. Variants in DENND1A are associated with polycystic ovary syndrome in women of European ancestry. J Clin Endocrinol Metab 2012;97(7):E1342–7.
14. Goodarzi MO, Jones MR, Li X, et al. Replication of association of DENND1A and THADA variants with polycystic ovary syndrome in European cohorts. J Med Genet 2012;49(2):90–5.

15. Brower MA, Jones MR, Rotter JI, et al. Further investigation in Europeans of susceptibility variants for polycystic ovary syndrome discovered in genome-wide association studies of Chinese individuals. J Clin Endocrinol Metab 2014;100(1): E182–6.

16. Louwers YV, Stolk L, Uitterlinden AG, et al. Cross-ethnic meta-analysis of genetic variants for polycystic ovary syndrome. J Clin Endocrinol Metab 2013;98(12): E2006–12.

17. Day FR, Hinds DA, Tung JY, et al. Causal mechanisms and balancing selection inferred from genetic associations with polycystic ovary syndrome. Nat Commun 2015;6:8464.

18. Hayes MG, Urbanek M, Ehrmann DA, et al. Genome-wide association of polycystic ovary syndrome implicates alterations in gonadotropin secretion in European ancestry populations. Nat Commun 2015;6:7502.

19. Saxena R, Georgopoulos NA, Braaten TJ, et al. Han Chinese polycystic ovary syndrome risk variants in women of European ancestry: relationship to FSH levels and glucose tolerance. Hum Reprod 2015;30(6):1454–9.

20. Day F, Karaderi T, Jones MR, et al. Large-scale genome-wide meta-analysis of polycystic ovary syndrome suggests shared genetic architecture for different diagnosis criteria. PLoS Genet 2018;14(12):e1007813.

21. Castro V, Shen Y, Yu S, et al. Identification of subjects with polycystic ovary syndrome using electronic health records. Reprod Biol Endocrinol 2015;13(1):116.

22. Zhang YHK, Keaton JM, Hartzel DN, et al. A genome-wide association study of polycystic ovary syndrome identified from electronic health record. Am J Obstet Gynecol 2020;223(4):559.

23. Farh KK, Marson A, Zhu J, et al. Genetic and epigenetic fine mapping of causal autoimmune disease variants. Nature 2015;518(7539):337–43.

24. Monteiro AN, Freedman ML. Lessons from postgenome-wide association studies: functional analysis of cancer predisposition loci. J Intern Med 2013;274(5): 414–24.

25. Musunuru K, Strong A, Frank-Kamenetsky M, et al. From noncoding variant to phenotype via SORT1 at the 1p13 cholesterol locus. Nature 2010;466(7307): 714–9.

26. McCarroll SA, Huett A, Kuballa P, et al. Deletion polymorphism upstream of IRGM associated with altered IRGM expression and Crohn's disease. Nat Genet 2008; 40(9):1107–12.

27. Ruth KS, Campbell PJ, Chew S, et al. Genome-wide association study with 1000 genomes imputation identifies signals for nine sex hormone-related phenotypes. Eur J Hum Genet 2015;24(2):284–90.

28. Saxena R, Bjonnes AC, Georgopoulos NA, et al. Gene variants associated with age at menopause are also associated with polycystic ovary syndrome, gonadotrophins and ovarian volume. Hum Reprod 2015;30(7):1697–703.

29. Ward LD, Kellis M. HaploReg v4: systematic mining of putative causal variants, cell types, regulators and target genes for human complex traits and disease. Nucleic Acids Res 2016;44(D1):D877–81.

30. Rosenbloom KR, Sloan CA, Malladi VS, et al. ENCODE data in the UCSC genome browser: year 5 update. Nucleic Acids Res 2013;41(Database issue):D56–63.

31. Ruf-Zamojski F, Zhang Z, Zamojski M, et al. Single nucleus multi-omics regulatory atlas of the murine pituitary. bioRxiv 2020. https://doi.org/10.1101/2020.06.06. 138024.

32. Paul P, van den Hoorn T, Jongsma ML, et al. A Genome-wide multidimensional RNAi screen reveals pathways controlling MHC class II antigen presentation. Cell 2011;145(2):268–83.

33. Mutlu B, Chen HM, Moresco JJ, et al. Regulated nuclear accumulation of a histone methyltransferase times the onset of heterochromatin formation in C. elegans embryos. Sci Adv 2018;4(8):eaat6224.

34. Fortin J, Boehm U, Deng CX, et al. Follicle-stimulating hormone synthesis and fertility depend on SMAD4 and FOXL2. FASEB J 2014;28(8):3396–410.

35. Abel MH, Widen A, Wang X, et al. Pituitary gonadotrophic hormone synthesis, secretion, subunit gene expression and cell structure in normal and follicle-stimulating hormone beta knockout, follicle-stimulating hormone receptor knockout, luteinising hormone receptor knockout, hypogonadal and ovariectom-ised female mice. J Neuroendocrinol 2014;26(11):785–95.

36. Ruth KS, Day FR, Tyrrell J, et al. Using human genetics to understand the disease impacts of testosterone in men and women. Nat Med 2020;26(2):252–8.

37. McAllister JM, Modi B, Miller BA, et al. Overexpression of a DENND1A isoform produces a polycystic ovary syndrome theca phenotype. Proc Natl Acad Sci U S A 2014;111(15):E1519–27.

38. Shi J, Gao Q, Cao Y, et al. Dennd1a, a susceptibility gene for polycystic ovary syndrome, is essential for mouse embryogenesis. Dev Dyn 2019;248(5):351–62.

39. Teves ME, Modi BP, Kulkarni R, et al. Human DENND1A.V2 Drives Cyp17a1 expression and androgen production in mouse ovaries and adrenals. Int J Mol Sci 2020;21(7):2545.

40. Gray R, Wheatley K. How to avoid bias when comparing bone marrow transplantation with chemotherapy. Bone Marrow Transplant 1991;7(Suppl 3):9–12.

41. Carey AH, Chan KL, Short F, et al. Evidence for a single gene effect causing polycystic ovaries and male pattern baldness. Clin Endocrinol 1993;38(6):653–8.

42. Brower MA, Hai Y, Jones MR, et al. Bidirectional Mendelian randomization to explore the causal relationships between body mass index and polycystic ovary syndrome. Hum Reprod 2019;34(1):127–36.

43. Khera AV, Chaffin M, Aragam KG, et al. Genome-wide polygenic scores for common diseases identify individuals with risk equivalent to monogenic mutations. Nat Genet 2018;50(9):1219–24.

44. Joo YY, Actkins K, Pacheco JA, et al. A polygenic and phenotypic risk prediction for polycystic ovary syndrome evaluated by phenome-wide association studies. J Clin Endocrinol Metab 2020;105(6):1918–36.

45. Hollands GJ, Griffin SJ, Sutton S, et al. The impact of communicating genetic risks of disease on risk-reducing health behaviour: systematic review with meta-analysis. BMJ 2016;352:i1102.

46. Srouji SS, Pagan YL, D'Amato F, et al. Pharmacokinetic factors contribute to the inverse relationship between luteinizing hormone and body mass index in polycystic ovarian syndrome. J Clin Endocrinol Metab 2007;92(4):1347–52.

47. Legro RS, Barnhart HX, Schlaff WD, et al. Ovulatory response to treatment of polycystic ovary syndrome is associated with a polymorphism in the STK11 gene. J Clin Endocrinol Metab 2008;93(3):792–800.

48. Kiddy DS, Hamilton-Fairley D, Bush A, et al. Improvement in endocrine and ovarian function during dietary treatment of obese women with polycystic ovary syndrome. Clin Endocrinol 1992;36(1):105–11.

49. Flannick J, Mercader JM, Fuchsberger C, et al. Exome sequencing of 20,791 cases of type 2 diabetes and 24,440 controls. Nature 2019;570(7759):71–6.

50. Murphy MK, Hall JE, Adams JM, et al. Polycystic ovarian morphology in normal women does not predict the development of polycystic ovary syndrome. J Clin Endocrinol Metab 2006;91(10):3878–84.
51. Lindheim L, Bashir M, Munzker J, et al. Alterations in Gut Microbiome Composition and barrier function are associated with reproductive and metabolic defects in women with polycystic ovary syndrome (PCOS): a pilot study. PloS one 2017; 12(1):e0168390.
52. Peng Y, Zhang W, Yang P, et al. ERBB4 confers risk for polycystic ovary syndrome in Han Chinese. Sci Rep 2017;7:42000.
53. Tian Y, Zhao H, Chen H, et al. Variants in FSHB are associated with polycystic ovary syndrome and luteinizing hormone level in Han Chinese women. J Clin Endocrinol Metab 2016;101(5):2178–84.

Cardiometabolic Risk in Polycystic Ovary Syndrome
Current Guidelines

Laura G. Cooney, MD[a], Anuja Dokras, MD, PhD[b],*

KEYWORDS

- PCOS • Metabolic risk • Screening • Diabetes • Cardiovascular disease

KEY POINTS

- Women with polycystic ovary syndrome (PCOS) are at increased risk of obesity, impaired glucose tolerance, diabetes, dyslipidemia, hypertension, metabolic syndrome, venous thromboembolism, and subclinical atherosclerosis compared with women without POCS.
- Women with PCOS should be screened for these conditions at the time of diagnosis, and future screening should occur on a regular basis at intervals, depending on results and baseline risk.
- Despite the increased risk of traditional cardiovascular risk factors in women with PCOS, the true risk of cardiovascular events, such as myocardial infarction or stroke, in women with PCOS in unknown, although accumulating data suggest the potential for an association.

INTRODUCTION

Polycystic ovary syndrome (PCOS) is a complex endocrine disorder affecting 6% to 10% of women[1,2] and is associated with metabolic, reproductive, and psychological implications. Although the definition centers around 3 features—oligomenorrhea, clinical or biochemical signs of hyperandrogenism, and polycystic ovaries on ultrasound—it is important for clinicians to counsel patients regarding the long-term health risks and the need for early screening and management. The metabolic complications of PCOS are numerous, including overweight/obesity, impaired glucose tolerance (IGT) and diabetes, dyslipidemia, hypertension (HTN), and metabolic syndrome (MetS). Even more concerning is the potential for subclinical atherosclerosis and cardiovascular events, including myocardial infarction (MI) and stroke. This article's objective is to outline the evidence for metabolic and cardiovascular comorbidities and discuss screening recommendations.

[a] Department of Obstetrics and Gynecology, University of Wisconsin, Generations Fertility Care, 2365 Deming Way, Middleton, WI 53562, USA; [b] Department of Obstetrics and Gynecology, University of Pennsylvania, Penn Fertility Care, 3701 Market Street, Suite 800, Philadelphia, PA 19085, USA
* Corresponding author.
E-mail address: Adokras@pennmedicine.upenn.edu

Endocrinol Metab Clin N Am 50 (2021) 83–95
https://doi.org/10.1016/j.ecl.2020.11.001
0889-8529/21/© 2020 Elsevier Inc. All rights reserved.

OVERWEIGHT/OBESITY
Extent of the Problem

Approximately 60% of women with PCOS are obese,[3] and this risk appears to have a genetic predisposition.[4] Not only does obesity increase the risk of other metabolic complications associated with PCOS, such as dyslipidemia, type 2 diabetes mellitus (DM), HTN, and pregnancy complications, such as preeclampsia and gestational diabetes, but also it is one of the most common characteristics of PCOS that is cited by patients as a major concern.[5] Obesity also is related to increased risk of eating disorders, anxiety, and depression in women with PCOS.[6,7] Central obesity, often found in women with PCOS,[3] is known to be associated with more severe metabolic disturbances.[8]

There is a bidirectional relationship between PCOS and weight gain: women with PCOS are more likely to gain weight over time and weight gain predisposes to the risk of manifesting PCOS.[9,10] The risk of obesity varies by race, with white women having a higher odds of obesity compared with Asians (10.8-fold vs 2.3-fold, respectively; $P<.001$).[3] The risks for obesity and central obesity were similar irrespective of diagnostic criteria,[3] however, higher in the hyperandrogenic (HA) phenotypes (40% vs 11%, respectively; $P<.001$).[11] Both adolescents with PCOS[3] and older women with PCOS have increased risk of obesity.[12]

Screening Recommendations

Because weight gain in women with PCOS often starts in adolescence, early awareness of this risk and close monitoring are paramount in helping decrease weight gain trajectories. International guidelines recommend that women with PCOS should be monitored for weight changes every 6 months to 12 months (**Table 1**).[13,14] Given the association between negative body image and low self-esteem, it is important for providers to be tactful in discussing the risk of weight gain and obesity and participate in shared decision making about the frequency and manner of screening.

IMPAIRED GLUCOSE TOLERANCE AND TYPE 2 DIABETES MELLITUS
Extent of the Problem

Women with PCOS have increased risks of IGT and type 2 DM (odds ratio [OR] 3.26; 95% CI, 2.17–4.90; and OR 2.87; 95% CI, 1.44–5.72, respectively; meta-analysis of 40 studies).[15] Women living in the Asian subcontinent (5.2 fold) and North/South Americans (4.4 fold) had the highest risk of IGT, whereas the risk was moderate in Europe (2.6 fold). Similar ethnic distributions and risks were seen when evaluating for the risk of DM.[15] US studies show that Hispanic and black women have higher degrees of insulin resistance compared with non-Hispanic whites.[16,17] The increased prevalence of IGT was noted in body mass index (BMI)-matched (2.1 fold), non–BMI-matched (4.8 fold), lean-matched (4.4 fold), and overweight or obese–matched groups (2.5 fold).[15] On the contrary, Kakoly and colleagues[15] did not find an increased risk of DM in subgroups matched on BMI (OR 1.13; 95% CI, 0.83–1.54; 7 studies), perhaps due to the small numbers in this subanalysis and a young mean age (30 years). Another study reported a higher risk of DM in nonobese women with PCOS compared with nonobese controls (OR 1.5; 95% CI, 1.1–2.0; $P = .007$; 5 studies), although they had less stringent inclusion criteria for the diagnosis of PCOS in their meta-analysis.[18]

Two longitudinal studies[19,20] conducted over 10 years found a higher incidence of DM in the PCOS cohort compared with controls. They each had limitations, however, including self-report of PCOS diagnosis[19] or use of administrative codes for PCOS

Table 1
Screening recommendations for women with polycystic ovary syndrome

Metabolic Morbidity	Who Should be Screened?	Screening Recommendations	Screening Intervals	Special Considerations
Obesity	All women at time of PCOS diagnosis	• Weight and height to calculate BMI • Ideally, waist circumference	Every 6–12 mo	
IGT, type 2 DM	All women at time of PCOS diagnosis	• Fasting glucose or HbA$_{1c}$ in low risk women or • OTT in higher risk women (BMI >25 kg/m^2 or in Asians >23 kg/m^2, history of abnormal glucose tolerance, or family history of diabetes)	Every 1–3 y based on risk factors for DM	• An OGTT should be offered in all women with PCOS who are planning pregnancy or seeking fertility treatment. • If not performed preconception, an OGTT should be offered at <20 wk gestation and all women with PCOS should have an OGTT at 24–28 wk gestation.
Dyslipidemia	All women (regardless of weight) after age 20^3 Adolescents who are overweight or obese at time of PCOS diagnosis	• Fasting lipid profile (cholesterol, LDL, HDL, and TG levels)	Repeat measurement should be guided based on results or global CVD risk. ACC/AHA guidelines recommend at least every 4–6 y	
HTN	All women at time of diagnosis	• Blood pressure	Annually or more frequently based on global CVD risk.	

Data from Teede HJ, Misso ML, Costello MF; et al. Recommendations from the international evidence-based guideline for the assessment and management of polycystic ovary syndrome. *Fertil Steril.* 2018; 110(3):364-379 and Arnett DK, Blumenthal RS, Albert MA, et al. 2019 ACC/AHA Guideline on the Primary Prevention of Cardiovascular Disease. *A Report of the American College of Cardiology/American Heart Association Task Force on Clinical Practice Guidelines.* 2019;74(10):e177-e232.

and/or hirsutism.[20] Population-based studies also have shown higher rates of DM in women with PCOS,[21–24] some of which also adjusted for BMI.[22,23]

A large cross-sectional study found higher rates of insulin resistance in the HA PCOS phenotypes but no difference in rates of hyperglycemia in PCOS phenotypes.[11] Similarly, a recent large cross-sectional study of PCOS identified from a hospital-based cohort in China (N = 2436) showed that all 4 Rotterdam phenotypes had a similar prevalence of DM.[25]

There are few data on prevalence of IGT and DM in adolescents. The meta-analysis by Kakoly and colleagues[15] included 7 studies with subjects less than 20 years, 5 of which were higher quality. Three showed a nonsignificant increase in IGT in adolescents with PCOS and 2 had no cases of IGT/DM in either the PCOS or the control group. The small number of subjects in each study limits the ability to draw firm conclusions in this age group.[15] In a systematic review, the authors' group previously reported that 7 of 10 studies reported an increased prevalence of IGT and/or DM in women with PCOS over age 40 years.[12] More recently, 2 longitudinal studies have examined the risk of DM in older women; 1 showed an increased risk (mean age at follow-up: 52 years),[26] but the other reported an increased risk in younger (<40 years), but not older, women with PCOS.[27]

Overall, the data support that reproductive-aged and perimenopausal/menopausal women with PCOS are at an increased risk of IGT and DM. Furthermore, cross-sectional studies demonstrate the increased risk of IGT is independent of obesity. Although cross-sectional studies do not show an increased risk of DM independent of BMI, multiple larger population-based and longitudinal studies have demonstrated an increased risk of DM even after adjusting for BMI.[19,22,23,27] Future studies should focus on evaluation of the risk of IGT/DM in adolescents.

Screening Recommendations

Given the increased prevalence of IGT and DM in women with PCOS, close monitoring is necessary. In the general population, those with IGT at baseline develop DM at a yearly rate of 5.7%.[28] In a study of women with PCOS in Thailand (N = 400), BMI greater than 23 kg/m^2 and impaired fasting glucose at baseline were 2 important predictors in the development of DM after 5 years of follow-up.[29] The international guidelines recommend screening for IGT/DM at time of diagnosis and every 1 year to 3 years thereafter based on risk (see **Table 1**). Screening for low risk women can consist of a fasting glucose or hemoglobin (Hb) A_{1c}, but higher risk women (BMI >25 kg/m^2 or, in Asians, BMI >23 kg/m^2; history of IGT;or family history of DM) and women who are seeking pregnancy or fertility treatment should be offered an oral glucose tolerance test (OGTT).[14]

Although discussion of treatment is beyond the scope of this article, the guidelines recommend starting metformin, in addition to lifestyle recommendations, in women with PCOS who have IGT or DM. The guidelines also suggest considering the use of metformin in women with PCOS with BMI greater than or equal to 25 kg/m^2 without IGT/DM,[14] Metformin has been shown to decrease progression from IGT to DM in the general population[30] and to decrease BMI in women with PCOS.[31]

DYSLIPIDEMIA
Extent of the Problem

In a meta-analysis of 30 studies,[32] women with PCOS were found to have a higher mean serum low-density lipoprotein (LDL) cholesterol (LDL-C), non–high-density lipoprotein (HDL) cholesterol (non–HDL-C), and triglyceride (TG) levels and lower HDL-C levels compared with women without PCOS, although overall differences were small (ie standardized mean difference [SMD] between groups: 12 mg/dL for LDL-C), raising the question of clinical significance. In studies that matched on BMI, the association between PCOS and elevated LDL-C and non–HDL-C persisted.[32] The HA phenotype is associated with a higher risk of dyslipidemia with low HDL-C in women with HA-PCOS.[11] Among women with PCOS, non-Hispanic black women may have a lower prevalence of dyslipidemia compared with both Hispanics and non-Hispanic whites.[16,17] In a meta-analysis in adolescents with PCOS, there were no significant differences in TG and HDL-C levels, however. this study was limited by low numbers (6 of 7 studies included <70 PCOS subjects).[33] A few large studies examining the risk of dyslipidemia in older women (>40) also have shown an association with PCOS.[12] Future studies should assess the prevalence of dyslipidemia in women of all ages independent of BMI.

Screening Recommendations

The American College of Cardiology/American Heart Association (ACC/AHA) guidelines recommend screening for lipid disorders in all patients aged 20 years to 45 years every 4 years to 6 years.[34] International PCOS guidelines recommend a fasting lipid profile at the time of PCOS diagnosis in overweight and obese women regardless of age (see **Table 1**). These guidelines suggest that the interval for repeat testing should be based on results of initial testing and global risk of cardiovascular disease (CVD).

HYPERTENSION
Extent of the Problem

In a meta-analysis,[35] the overall pooled prevalence of HTN was higher in women with PCOS compared with controls (15% vs 9%, respectively). When evaluating non–population-based studies separated by age, this association was seen only in studies of reproductive-aged women (OR 1.5; 95% CI, 1.2–1.8) and not menopausal women (OR 1.5; 95% CI, 0.91–2.3), although there were fewer studies of older women. The investigators did not report findings adjusted for BMI.[35] Daan and colleagues[11] found a higher prevalence of HTN in the HA PCOS phenotypes in unadjusted but not adjusted analysis. Among women with PCOS, non-Hispanic white women have the lowest prevalence of HTN.[16,17]

Two longitudinal studies also did not report significant differences in HTN[36,37] In adolescents with PCOS a higher systolic blood pressure but not diastolic blood pressure was reported compared with controls (SMD 5.0; 95% CI, 1.3–8.7; and SMD 3.5; 95% CI, 0.5–8.6, respectively).[33]

In summary, the reported prevalence of HTN varies considerably. Most studies do not show a continued risk of HTN, independent of BMI, after menopause.[12] and data in adolescents are limfited.

Screening Recommendations

International guidelines recommend that all women with PCOS have blood pressure measured annually (see **Table 1**).[14]

METABOLIC SYNDROME
Extent of the Problem

MetS is a cluster of metabolic disturbances, including central obesity, hyperglycemia/insulin resistance, dyslipidemia, and HTN. In young adults with PCOS, the mean prevalence of MetS is estimated to be 30% (95% CI, 27–33; 46 studies)[38] with a 2-fold to 3-

fold increased odds of MetS compared with controls.[18,39–41] In sensitivity analyses, Lim and colleagues[40] demonstrated that this increased prevalence persisted in BMI-matched studies (OR 1.8; 95% CI, 1.3–2.3) and in overweight or obese women (OR 1.88%; 95% CI, 1.16–3.04) but not in lean women (OR 1.45; 95% CI, 0.35–6.12). When evaluating geographic differences, all regions had increased odds of MetS in women with PCOS (Europe: 2.6-fold, Americas: 5.2-fold, Asia: 3.5-fold; and Australia and New Zealand: 3.6-fold). These studies on phenotype are limited, however, by not controlling for BMI. Hispanic women with PCOS had a higher prevalence of MetS compared with non-Hispanic black women in some[16] but not all studies.[17] Several meta-analyses have suggested a relationship between PCOS phenotype and prevalence of MetS.[39,40,42] In a meta-analysis specifically evaluating phenotype, Yang and colleagues[42] found increased odds of MetS in women with HA phenotype compared with women with PCOS without HA (OR 2.21; 95% CI, 1.88–2.59). The risk of MetS in older women with PCOS is less clear. The prevalence of MetS increases with use of OCPs in overweight/obese women with PCOS and can be mitigated by lifestyle modifications.[43]

In summary, the risk of MetS clearly is higher in adolescent and reproductive-aged women with PCOS in several regions of the world.

Screening Recommendations

MetS is associated with an increased risk of DM, cardiovascular disorders, coronary heart disease, stroke, and mortality[44]; thus, as with its individual components, appropriate screening and diagnosis are paramount.[45] Frequent assessment in overweight/obese women with PCOS prescribed combined hormonal contraceptives allows early detection of metabolic risk factors.

CARDIOVASCULAR DISEASE: SUBCLINICAL ATHEROSCLEROSIS
Extent of the Problem

In addition to the traditional risk factors for CVD, discussed previously, evidence of subclinical atherosclerosis has been shown associated with CVD events, including stroke and MI. Common methods of evaluating subclinical atherosclerosis are measuring carotid artery intima media thickness (C-IMT) endothelia dysfunction, measured by comparing changes in arterial flow-mediated dilation (FMD); and coronary artery calcium (CAC) scores, which are measured with the use of cardiac computerized tomography or magnetic resonance imaging. In the general population, increases in C-IMT, lower FMD, and higher CAC scores are associated with increased risks of CVD events.[46–50]

A meta-analyses showed that women with PCOS have a higher C-IMT compared with controls (SMD 0.072 mm; 95% CI, 0.040–0.105; P<.0001; meta-analysis of 19 studies).[51] In the general population, for every 0.1-mm incremental increase in mean C-IMT, the hazard of stroke increases by 18% and the hazard of MI increases by 15%.[47] In another meta-analysis, women with PCOS had a 3.4% lower pooled mean FMD (95% CI, 1.9–4.9; meta-analysis of 21 studies) than control women. Their results remained significant after matching on age and BM.[52] Most women in these studies were in the second or third decade of life, suggesting that evidence for subclinical atherosclerosis can be detected at a young age. CAC scores also have been reported to be higher in some small studies of young women with PCOS[53,54] but not in others.[55]

An evaluation of phenotypic differences in risk of atherosclerosis is limited because none of the meta-analyses evaluated phenotype. Also, no differences based on race are reported.[17] Studies on subclinical atherosclerosis in older women with PCOS are mixed, with most not showing a higher prevalence.[12] This leaves the question open as to whether women with PCOS potentially develop atherosclerosis at a younger age than women without PCOS but that women without PCOS catch-up, such that at older ages there is no longer a difference.

In summary, younger women have an increased prevalence of subclinical atherosclerosis, but this risk is unclear past the reproductive years. Longitudinal studies with well-phenotyped women with PCOS are needed to evaluate persistent risk in the perimenopause and beyond.

Screening Recommendations

There are no specific recommendations for screening for evidence of subclinical atherosclerosis in women with PCOS. CAC scores have not been incorporated into current CVD risk assessment algorithms although they may improve risk stratification.

CARDIOVASCULAR DISEASE: VENOUS THROMBOEMBOLISM
Extent of the Problem

Women with PCOS have risk factors for venous thromboembolism (VTE), including obesity, DM, dyslipidemia, and HTN. In addition, first-line treatment of PCOS is combined oral contraceptive pills (COCs), which also can increase the risk of VTE. A meta-analysis of 3 studies (mean age 30 years), which controlled for BMI, demonstrated that women with PCOS had an increased risk of VTE compared with controls (adjusted OR 1.9; 95% CI, 1.6–2.2). These population-based studies used *International Classification of Diseases, Ninth Revision (ICD-9)* codes for obesity to control for BMI using either propensity scores or regression models; however, prevalence of obesity in the populations were low (1%–13%), suggesting there could be residual confounding and underestimation of the impact of BMI on VTE risk.

Data are mixed on the effect of concurrent COC use on VTE risk, with 1 study showing increased risk for VTE in women with PCOS taking COCs[56] and another showing a decreased risk[57] Given the young age of these populations, the absolute risk of VTE among women with PCOS is low, ranging from 6.3 to 28.3 per 10,000 person years.[56–58]

Screening Recommendations

International guidelines for use of COCs in women with PCOS recommend use of the lowest effective estrogen doses (such as 20–30 µg of ethinyl estradiol or equivalent)[14] to minimize risk of VTE.

CARDIOVASCULAR DISEASE EVENTS: MYOCARDIAL INFARCTION OR STROKE
Extent of the Problem

Studies in women with PCOS examining CVD outcomes use the following endpoints: CV death, nonfatal MI, nonfatal stroke, and hospitalization for unstable angina.[59] There are several limitations in the current studies. First, CV events are rare in young women, such that large numbers of women are needed to have sufficient power to detect differences at a young age. Second, diagnosis of PCOS is difficult to establish in older women and is subject to recall bias, because symptoms, such as menstrual irregularity and hirsutism, improve with age.[60,61] Despite these limitations, there are multiple meta-analyses attempting to evaluate the association between PCOS and CV events.[62–64] Unfortunately, included studies had limitations, such as a presumed diagnosis of PCOS based on menstrual irregularity only[37,65] or inclusion of non-Rotterdam criteria, such as infertility, history of miscarriage, obesity, or insulin resistance.[66,67] A meta-analysis performed for the international guidelines attempted to include only quality studies[14] and did not find a difference in risk of MI (OR 1.21; 95% CI, 0.68–2.14; P = 0.5; 3 studies), stroke (OR 1.64; 95% CI, 0.92–2.93; P = 0.1; 4 studies), CVD-related death (OR 1.81; 95% CI, 0.55–5.88; P = .3; 2 studies), or coronary artery/heart disease (OR 2.44; 95% CI, 0.88–6.74; P = .09; 2 studies).[14] They did include a study,[68] however, where all of the women with PCOS had a history of a wedge resection. It is unclear how this would bias their results because perhaps the women in this study had a more severe PCOS phenotype necessitating treatment or, by contrary, the surgery may have resulted in subsequent improvement in androgens or oligomenorrhea, thereby mitigating their future CVD risks. The 2 other studies had very low numbers (<35 women with PCOS).[24,69]

Given the small numbers of subjects and young age of participants (mean ages of women in the 2 largest studies included in this analysis were <40 years at follow-up) and the absolute risk of a CVD event being very low in this population, it is likely that these studies are underpowered. Thus, the question of a true association between PCOS and CVD is unanswered by these meta-analyses of cross-sectional studies.

A study by Mani and colleagues,[70] not included in the meta-analysis, discussed previously, compared women with PCOS (N = 2301) diagnosed in an endocrinology clinic to age-matched control women. They reported that women with PCOS had higher odds of MI than controls in all age groups greater than age 45 years.[70] Most meta-analyses did not include any registry or population-based studies given the limitations of using *ICD-9* codes. In the absence of definitive data from other sources, however, population-based studies can be helpful in evaluating the risk of CV events because they allow for large sample sizes, long follow-up times, and, in some cases, adjusting for confounders, such as BMI.

There are 6 population-based studies evaluating CVD events in women with PCOS, some of which followed women for more than 10 years. Four showed increased odds of CVD events in women with PCOS, 3 of which adjusted for BMI.[21,22,71,72] These studies are limited by potential inaccuracies with PCOS diagnosis[71,72] or inclusion of only hospitalized women.[22] Two studies did not show increased rates of VD events; however, the mean ages were less than 30 years.[23,73] There is 1 meta-analysis evaluating just population studies, which found a higher odds of CV events and mortality due to CV events in women with PCOS (OR 1.8; 95% CI, 1.5–2.1; and OR 1.8; 95% CI, 1.5–2.1; respectively)[64]

Taken together, there is a suggestion of an increased prevalence of CVD events in women with PCOS when evaluating a combination of cross-sectional, cohort, and population-based studies, although most studies have limitations. The ideal study would include a large cohort of reproductive-age women with well characterized PCOS phenotype and follow-up data for several decades. Long duration of follow-up is needed, given the low prevalence of CV events in premenopausal women.

Screening Recommendations

Clinicians can use the ACC/AHA calculator for computing the 10-year risk of an atherosclerotic CVD event, in women over the age of 40.

SUMMARY

In conclusion, all women with PCOS need to be counseled regarding their increased risks of obesity, IGT, DM, dyslipidemia, HTN, MetS, VTE, and subclinical atherosclerosis. Screening for these conditions should be conducted at the time of diagnosis and repeated based on risk factors to facilitate early identification and treatment of metabolic conditions. Due to several limitations in the current studies, it is not clear if the risks observed in the reproductive years persist into the perimenopause and menopausal period. Data support that the risk of both obesity and DM continues at older ages, confirming the need for frequent screening. Management of PCOS should be comprehensive and include a multidisciplinary model of care to treat comorbidities associated with PCOS, including cardiometabolic, psychological, dermatologic, and infertility. Future studies should focus on better elucidating the risk of CVD in women with PCOS specifically in the postmenopausal years so that women can be counseled accurately. In the meantime, risk stratification should occur based on known risk factors for CVD and prediction models created for the general population.

CLINICS CARE POINTS

- Adolescents and women with PCOS are at an increased risk for obesity and should be monitored for weight gain and counseled regarding weight management strategies.
- Reproductive-aged women with PCOS are at an increased risk for IGT and diabetes and should be screened at the time of diagnosis irrespective of their weight; follow-up screening can occur at regular intervals based on other risk factors.
- The prevalence of metabolic risk factors appears to be higher in the HA PCOS phenotypes as defined by the Rotterdam criteria.
- Risk of VTE in women with PCOS can be minimized by starting with oral contraceptives that contain the lowest effective estrogen doses.
- It is important to be aware of early screening recommendations as for many conditions often starts at younger ages than recommended for the general population.

DISCLOSURES

The authors have nothing to disclose.

REFERENCES

1. Bozdag G, Mumusoglu S, Zengin D, et al. The prevalence and phenotypic features of polycystic ovary syndrome: a systematic review and meta-analysis. Hum Reprod 2016;31(12):2841–55.
2. Lizneva D, Suturina L, Walker W, et al. Criteria, prevalence, and phenotypes of polycystic ovary syndrome. Fertil Steril 2016;106(1):6–15.
3. Lim SS, Davies MJ, Norman RJ, et al. Overweight, obesity and central obesity in women with polycystic ovary syndrome: a systematic review and meta-analysis. Hum Reprod Update 2012;18(6):618–37.
4. Day FR, Hinds DA, Tung JY, et al. Causal mechanisms and balancing selection inferred from genetic associations with polycystic ovary syndrome. Nat Commun 2015;6:8464.
5. Gibson-Helm M, Teede H, Dunaif A, et al. Delayed diagnosis and a lack of information associated with dissatisfaction in women with polycystic ovary syndrome. J Clin Endocrinol Metab 2017;102(2):604–12.
6. Lee I, Cooney LG, Saini S, et al. Increased risk of disordered eating in polycystic ovary syndrome. Fertil Steril 2017;107(3):796–802.

7. Cooney LG, Lee I, Sammel MD, et al. High prevalence of moderate and severe depressive and anxiety symptoms in polycystic ovary syndrome: a systematic review and meta-analysis. Hum Reprod 2017;32(5):1075–91.

8. Pasquali R. Obesity and androgens: facts and perspectives. Fertil Steril 2006; 85(5):1319–40.

9. Ollila MM, Piltonen T, Puukka K, et al. Weight gain and dyslipidemia in early adulthood associate with polycystic ovary syndrome: prospective cohort study. J Clin Endocrinol Metab 2016;101(2):739–47.

10. Yildiz BO, Knochenhauer ES, Azziz R. Impact of obesity on the risk for polycystic ovary syndrome. J Clin Endocrinol Metab 2008;93(1):162–8.

11. Daan NM, Louwers YV, Koster MP, et al. Cardiovascular and metabolic profiles amongst different polycystic ovary syndrome phenotypes: who is really at risk? Fertil Steril 2014;102(5):1444–51.e1443.

12. Laura G, Cooney M, Anuja Dokras. Beyond fertility: polycystic ovary syndrome and long-term health. Fertil Steril 2018;110(5):794–809.

13. Teede HJ, Misso ML, Costello MF, et al. Recommendations from the international evidence-based guideline for the assessment and management of polycystic ovary syndrome. Fertil Steril 2018;110(3):364–79.

14. International evidence-based guideline for the assessment and management of polycystic ovary syndrome. Monash University. 2018. Available at: https://www. monash.edu/__data/assets/pdf_file/0004/1412644/PCOS-Evidence-Based-Guideline.pdf. Accessed April 22, 2020.

15. Kakoly NS, Khomami MB, Joham AE, et al. Ethnicity, obesity and the prevalence of impaired glucose tolerance and type 2 diabetes in PCOS: a systematic review and meta-regression. Hum Reprod Update 2018;24(4):455–67.

16. Engmann L, Jin S, Sun F, et al. Racial and ethnic differences in the polycystic ovary syndrome metabolic phenotype. Am J Obstet Gynecol 2017;216(5). 493.e491-493.e413.

17. Chang AY, Oshiro J, Ayers C, et al. Influence of race/ethnicity on cardiovascular risk factors in polycystic ovary syndrome, the Dallas Heart Study. Clin Endocrinol 2016;85(1):92–9.

18. Zhu S, Zhang B, Jiang X, et al. Metabolic disturbances in non-obese women with polycystic ovary syndrome: a systematic review and meta-analysis. Fertil Steril 2019;111(1):168–77.

19. Kakoly NS, Earnest A, Teede HJ, et al. The impact of obesity on the incidence of type 2 diabetes among women with polycystic ovary syndrome. Diabetes Care 2019;42(4):560–7.

20. Rubin KH, Glintborg D, Nybo M, et al. Development and risk factors of type 2 diabetes in a nationwide population of women with polycystic ovary syndrome. J Clin Endocrinol Metab 2017;102(10):3848–57.

21. Ding DC, Tsai IJ, Wang JH, et al. Coronary artery disease risk in young women with polycystic ovary syndrome. Oncotarget 2018;9(9):8756–64.

22. Hart R, Doherty DA. The potential implications of a PCOS diagnosis on a woman's long-term health using data linkage. J Clin Endocrinol Metab 2015;100(3):911–9.

23. Lo JC, Feigenbaum SL, Yang J, et al. Epidemiology and adverse cardiovascular risk profile of diagnosed polycystic ovary syndrome. J Clin Endocrinol Metab 2006;91(4):1357–63.

24. Schmidt J, Landin-Wilhelmsen K, Brannstrom M, et al. Cardiovascular disease and risk factors in PCOS women of postmenopausal age: a 21-year controlled follow-up study. J Clin Endocrinol Metab 2011;96(12):3794–803.

25. Li H, Li L, Gu J, et al. Should all women with polycystic ovary syndrome be screened for metabolic parameters?: a hospital-based observational study. PLoS One 2016;11(11):e0167036.
26. Forslund M, Landin-Wilhelmsen K, Trimpou P, et al. Type 2 diabetes mellitus in women with polycystic ovary syndrome during a 24-year period: importance of obesity and abdominal fat distribution. Hum Reprod Open 2020;2020(1):hoz042.
27. Kazemi Jaliseh H, Ramezani Tehrani F, Behboudi-Gandevani S, et al. Polycystic ovary syndrome is a risk factor for diabetes and prediabetes in middle-aged but not elderly women: a long-term population-based follow-up study. Fertil Steril 2017;108(6):1078–84.
28. Edelstein SL, Knowler WC, Bain RP, et al. Predictors of progression from impaired glucose tolerance to NIDDM: an analysis of six prospective studies. Diabetes 1997;46(4):701–10.
29. Chantrapanichkul P, Indhavivadhana S, Wongwananuruk T, et al. Prevalence of type 2 diabetes mellitus compared between lean and overweight/obese patients with polycystic ovarian syndrome: a 5-year follow-up study. Arch Gynecol Obstet 2020;301(3):809–16.
30. Knowler WC, Barrett-Connor E, Fowler SE, et al. Reduction in the incidence of type 2 diabetes with lifestyle intervention or metformin. N Engl J Med 2002; 346(6):393–403.
31. Naderpoor N, Shorakae S, de Courten B, et al. Metformin and lifestyle modification in polycystic ovary syndrome: systematic review and meta-analysis. Hum Reprod Update 2015;21(5):560–74.
32. Wild RA, Rizzo M, Clifton S, et al. Lipid levels in polycystic ovary syndrome: systematic review and meta-analysis. Fertil Steril 2011;95(3):1073–9.e1071-1011.
33. Fazleen NE, Whittaker M, Mamun A. Risk of metabolic syndrome in adolescents with polycystic ovarian syndrome: a systematic review and meta-analysis. Diabetes Metab Syndr 2018;12(6):1083–90.
34. Arnett DK, Blumenthal RS, Albert MA, et al. 2019 ACC/AHA guideline on the primary prevention of cardiovascular disease. A report of the American college of cardiology/American heart association task force on clinical practice guidelines. Am Coll Cardiol 2019;74(10):e177–232.
35. Amiri M, Ramezani Tehrani F, Behboudi-Gandevani S, et al. Risk of hypertension in women with polycystic ovary syndrome: a systematic review, meta-analysis and meta-regression. Reprod Biol Endocrinol 2020;18(1):23.
36. Joham AE, Boyle JA, Zoungas S, et al. Hypertension in reproductive-aged women with polycystic ovary syndrome and association with obesity. Am J Hypertens 2015;28(7):847–51.
37. Wang ET, Cirillo PM, Vittinghoff E, et al. Menstrual irregularity and cardiovascular mortality. J Clin Endocrinol Metab 2011;96(1):E114–8.
38. Khorshidi A, Azami M, Tardeh S, et al. The prevalence of metabolic syndrome in patients with polycystic ovary syndrome: a systematic review and meta-analysis. Diabetes Metab Syndr 2019;13(4):2747–53.
39. Behboudi-Gandevani S, Amiri M, Bidhendi Yarandi R, et al. The risk of metabolic syndrome in polycystic ovary syndrome: a systematic review and meta-analysis. Clin Endocrinol (Oxf) 2018;88(2):169–84.
40. Lim SS, Kakoly NS, Tan JWJ, et al. Metabolic syndrome in polycystic ovary syndrome: a systematic review, meta-analysis and meta-regression. Obes Rev 2019; 20(2):339–52.

41. Otaghi M, Azami M, Khorshidi A, et al. The association between metabolic syndrome and polycystic ovary syndrome: a systematic review and meta-analysis. Diabetes Metab Syndr 2019;13(2):1481–9.
42. Yang R, Yang S, Li R, et al. Effects of hyperandrogenism on metabolic abnormalities in patients with polycystic ovary syndrome: a meta-analysis. Reprod Biol Endocrinol 2016;14(1):67.
43. Legro RS, Dodson WC, Kris-Etherton PM, et al. Randomized controlled trial of preconception interventions in infertile women with polycystic ovary syndrome. J Clin Endocrinol Metab 2015;100(11):4048–58.
44. Ford ES. The metabolic syndrome and mortality from cardiovascular disease and all-causes: findings from the national health and nutrition examination survey II mortality study. Atherosclerosis 2004;173(2):309–14.
45. Grundy SM, Cleeman JI, Daniels SR, et al. Diagnosis and management of the metabolic syndrome: an American heart association/national heart, lung, and blood institute scientific statement. Circulation 2005;112(17):2735–52.
46. Katakami N, Mita T, Gosho M, et al. Clinical utility of carotid ultrasonography in the prediction of cardiovascular events in patients with diabetes: a combined analysis of data obtained in five longitudinal studies. J Atheroscler Thromb 2018; 25(10):1053–66.
47. Lorenz MW, Markus HS, Bots ML, et al. Prediction of clinical cardiovascular events with carotid intima-media thickness: a systematic review and meta-analysis. Circulation 2007;115(4):459–67.
48. Shechter M, Shechter A, Koren-Morag N, et al. Usefulness of brachial artery flow-mediated dilation to predict long-term cardiovascular events in subjects without heart disease. Am J Cardiol 2014;113(1):162–7.
49. Detrano R, Guerci AD, Carr JJ, et al. Coronary calcium as a predictor of coronary events in four racial or ethnic groups. N Engl J Med 2008;358(13):1336–45.
50. Raggi P, Gongora MC, Gopal A, et al. Coronary artery calcium to predict all-cause mortality in elderly men and women. J Am Coll Cardiol 2008;52(1):17–23.
51. Meyer ML, Malek AM, Wild RA, et al. Carotid artery intima-media thickness in polycystic ovary syndrome: a systematic review and meta-analysis. Hum Reprod Update 2012;18(2):112–26.
52. Sprung VS, Atkinson G, Cuthbertson DJ, et al. Endothelial function measured using flow-mediated dilation in polycystic ovary syndrome: a meta-analysis of the observational studies. Clin Endocrinol (Oxf) 2013;78(3):438–46.
53. Shroff R, Kerchner A, Maifeld M, et al. Young obese women with polycystic ovary syndrome have evidence of early coronary atherosclerosis. J Clin Endocrinol Metab 2007;92(12):4609–14.
54. Talbott EO, Guzick DS, Sutton-Tyrrell K, et al. Evidence for association between polycystic ovary syndrome and premature carotid atherosclerosis in middle-aged women. Arterioscler Thromb Vasc Biol 2000;20(11):2414–21.
55. Christian RC, Dumesic DA, Behrenbeck T, et al. Prevalence and predictors of coronary artery calcification in women with polycystic ovary syndrome. J Clin Endocrinol Metab 2003;88(6):2562–8.
56. Bird ST, Hartzema AG, Brophy JM, et al. Risk of venous thromboembolism in women with polycystic ovary syndrome: a population-based matched cohort analysis. CMAJ 2013;185(2):E115–20.
57. Okoroh EM, Hooper WC, Atrash HK, et al. Is polycystic ovary syndrome another risk factor for venous thromboembolism? United States, 2003-2008. Am J Obstet Gynecol 2012;207(5):377.e1-8.

58. Gariani K, Hugon-Rodin J, Philippe J, et al. Association between polycystic ovary syndrome and venous thromboembolism: a systematic review and meta-analysis. Thromb Res 2020;185:102–8.
59. Hicks KA, Mahaffey KW, Mehran R, et al. 2017 Cardiovascular and stroke endpoint definitions for clinical trials. J Am Coll Cardiol 2018;71(9):1021–34.
60. Elting MW, Korsen TJ, Rekers-Mombarg LT, et al. Women with polycystic ovary syndrome gain regular menstrual cycles when ageing. Hum Reprod 2000; 15(1):24–8.
61. Winters SJ, Talbott E, Guzick DS, et al. Serum testosterone levels decrease in middle age in women with the polycystic ovary syndrome. Fertil Steril 2000; 73(4):724–9.
62. Zhao L, Zhu Z, Lou H, et al. Polycystic ovary syndrome (PCOS) and the risk of coronary heart disease (CHD): a meta-analysis. Oncotarget 2016;7(23): 33715–21.
63. Zhou Y, Wang X, Jiang Y, et al. Association between polycystic ovary syndrome and the risk of stroke and all-cause mortality: insights from a meta-analysis. Gynecol Endocrinol 2017;33(12):904–10.
64. Tehrani F, Ramezani, Amiri M, et al. Cardiovascular events among reproductive and menopausal age women with polycystic ovary syndrome: a systematic review and meta-analysis. Gynecol Endocrinol 2020;36(1):12–23.
65. Solomon CG, Hu FB, Dunaif A, et al. Menstrual cycle irregularity and risk for future cardiovascular disease. J Clin Endocrinol Metab 2002;87(5):2013–7.
66. Cheang KI, Nestler JE, Futterweit W. Risk of cardiovascular events in mothers of women with polycystic ovary syndrome. Endocr Pract 2008;14(9):1084–94.
67. Krentz AJ, von Muhlen D, Barrett-Connor E. Searching for polycystic ovary syndrome in postmenopausal women: evidence of a dose-effect association with prevalent cardiovascular disease. Menopause 2007;14(2):284–92.
68. Lunde O, Tanbo T. Polycystic ovary syndrome: a follow-up study on diabetes mellitus, cardiovascular disease and malignancy 15-25 years after ovarian wedge resection. Gynecol Endocrinol 2007;23(12):704–9.
69. Cibula D, Cifkova R, Fanta M, et al. Increased risk of non-insulin dependent diabetes mellitus, arterial hypertension and coronary artery disease in perimenopausal women with a history of the polycystic ovary syndrome. Hum Reprod 2000;15(4):785–9.
70. Mani H, Levy MJ, Davies MJ, et al. Diabetes and cardiovascular events in women with polycystic ovary syndrome: a 20-year retrospective cohort study. Clin Endocrinol (Oxf) 2013;78(6):926–34.
71. Glintborg D, Rubin KH, Nybo M, et al. Cardiovascular disease in a nationwide population of Danish women with polycystic ovary syndrome. Cardiovasc Diabetol 2018;17(1):37.
72. Okoroh EM, Boulet SL, George MG, et al. Assessing the intersection of cardiovascular disease, venous thromboembolism, and polycystic ovary syndrome. Thromb Res 2015;136(6):1165–8.
73. Sirmans SM, Parish RC, Blake S, et al. Epidemiology and comorbidities of polycystic ovary syndrome in an indigent population. J Investig Med 2014;62(6): 868–74.

Postmenopausal Hyperandrogenism
Evaluation and Treatment Strategies

Adnin Zaman, MD*, Micol S. Rothman, MD

KEYWORDS

- Postmenopausal • Hyperandrogenism • Virilization • Hyperthecosis
- Adrenal tumor(s) • Ovarian tumor(s)

KEY POINTS

- Postmenopausal hyperandrogenism can present with hirsutism and virilization.
- Changes are often mild and attributed to the normal aging process, but causes span both nontumorous and tumorous causes.
- This review details the evaluation and treatment of the unique differential of androgen excess in postmenopausal women.

INTRODUCTION

Postmenopausal androgen excess often occurs from the imbalance of rapidly decreasing ovarian estrogen with a relatively gradual decline in androgen secretion.[1] Symptoms of postmenopausal hyperandrogenism, such as increases in hirsutism or changes in hair patterns, are common and mild. Because these changes are attributed to the natural aging process with declines in sex-hormone binding globulin (SHBG) and subsequent increase in free androgen index,[2] clinicians often do not consider further clinical or biochemical evaluation. However, the development of rapid and true hirsutism, alopecia, and acne is rare and warrants further investigation. In the presence of virilizing signs, clinicians should consider an underlying malignancy.[3] A review of findings during the history, physical examination, and appropriate laboratory and radiologic evaluation will help guide in differentiating tumorous from nontumorous causes of postmenopausal hyperandrogenism, leading to optimal treatment strategies.

PRESENTING SIGNS AND SYMPTOMS

The diagnosis of postmenopausal androgen excess is based on patient presentation, thorough history, and physical examination. The most common complaints are facial

Division of Endocrinology, Metabolism and Diabetes, Department of Medicine, University of Colorado Anschutz Medical Campus, 12801 East 17th Avenue, MS 8106, Aurora, CO 80045, USA
* Corresponding author.
E-mail address: Adnin.Zaman@CUAnschutz.edu

Endocrinol Metab Clin N Am 50 (2021) 97–111
https://doi.org/10.1016/j.ecl.2020.12.002
0889-8529/21/© 2020 Elsevier Inc. All rights reserved.

endo.theclinics.com

or truncal hirsutism as well as loss of hair on the head. However, a detailed history is crucial in differentiating progressive hirsutism from true virilization. Hirsutism is defined as excessive terminal hair that appears in androgen-dependent areas (ie, in a male pattern) in women, such as on the chin, upper lip, and abdomen.[4] The Ferriman-Gallwey score has traditionally been used to quantify hirsutism in premenopausal women by assigning a score of 0 to 4 to describe hair patterns in the 9 body areas most sensitive to androgens,[5] but has not been validated for use in postmenopausal women. Virilization includes severe hirsutism along with male pattern balding, anabolic appearance or increased muscularity, lowering of the voice, and clitoromegaly (>1.5 × 2.5 cm).[4] Rapid progression of hirsutism along with virilization suggests severe hyperandrogenism and should trigger an evaluation for an androgen-secreting neoplasm.

A full menstrual history, including timing of menarche and menopause, prior irregular menses or premenopausal hyperandrogenism (ie, hirsutism, acne, and/or male pattern hair loss), should be obtained. The timing of acneiform lesions (ie, pubertal, perimenopausal, or sudden onset) may also be useful information. A personal history of headaches or visual disturbances may point to a pituitary disorder. A weight history, including timing of weight gain and loss, should also be elicited, particularly related to the onset of hirsutism and/or acne. A list of medications and supplements should be carefully obtained. A family history of endocrine disorders, hirsutism, or balding should also be recorded.[6]

Physical examination should include an evaluation of the extent of excess hair growth as well as acneiform lesions. Hair along the linea alba below the umbilicus is common in up to 20% of women. It is more concerning when hair is present on the upper chest and back and is associated with male pattern balding or clitoromegaly. Often, viewing pictures of the patient before symptom onset can be helpful. Because endocrinopathies can lead to postmenopausal hyperandrogenism, visual field testing for a pituitary tumor, evaluating for stigmata of hypercortisolism, and examining for galactorrhea are all indicated.

DIFFERENTIAL DIAGNOSIS

Broadly speaking, the differential diagnosis for postmenopausal hyperandrogenism can be divided into tumorous versus nontumorous causes. These causes and their presentations are outlined in **Table 1** and discussed later in detail.

The most common cause of hyperandrogenism in premenopausal women is the polycystic ovarian syndrome (PCOS), occurring in up to 12% of reproductive-aged women worldwide using the widely accepted 2003 Rotterdam Criteria.[7,8] The diagnosis of PCOS using the Rotterdam Criteria requires the presence of 2 of the 3 criteria after exclusion of other causes: oligomenorrhea/amenorrhea, clinical or biochemical hyperandrogenism, and polycystic morphology of ovaries on ultrasound. The 2009 Androgen Excess Society definition emphasizes the key role of hyperandrogenism and thus requires the presence clinical and/or biochemical hyperandrogenism in the setting of ovarian dysfunction (oligoanovulation and/or polycystic ovaries on ultrasound) after excluding related disorders.[9] The 1990 National Institutes of Health criteria are less commonly used and exclude ultrasound findings.[7,10] Although the signs and symptoms of PCOS are most notable during the reproductive years, diagnosis in the postmenopausal period may also occur. However, there is no established phenotype for PCOS in postmenopausal women.[11] Although signs and symptoms of hyperandrogenism may improve in PCOS patients after menopause, postmenopausal women with PCOS continue to have higher levels of both adrenal and ovarian

Table 1
Differential diagnosis and presentation of androgen excess in postmenopausal women

Diagnosis		Presentation in Postmenopausal Women
Nontumorous hyperandrogenism		
Endogenous causes		
Inherited disorders	PCOS	*Sx:* Premenopausal history of anovulatory cycles and hyperandrogenism *Data:* Elevated T and DHEAS
	NCCAH	*Sx:* Premenopausal history of anovulatory cycles and hyperandrogenism *Data:* Elevated 17-hydroxyprogesterone after ACTH stimulation
Obesity-induced hyperandrogenism		*Sx:* Progressive weight gain without return to baseline weight; normal menses until reaching threshold weight *Data:* Elevated T but otherwise normal laboratory tests and imaging studies
Hyperthecosis		*Sx:* Premenopausal history of anovulatory cycles and hyperandrogenism; postmenopausal virilization *Data:* Very high T, modest elevations in DHEAS; pelvic US with bilateral ovarian enlargement (≥ 10 cm^3)
Endocrinopathies	Cushing syndrome	*Sx:* Stigmata of glucocorticoid excess *Data:* Elevated cortisol on UFC, 1 mg DST, and/or salivary cortisol
	Hyperprolactinemia	*Sx:* Galactorrhea; headaches and/or visual disturbances with prolactinoma *Data:* Elevated serum prolactin level
	Acromegaly	*Sx:* Stigmata of GH excess *Data:* Elevated serum insulin-like growth factor-1, nonsuppressed GH with oral glucose tolerance testing

(continued on next page)

	Diagnosis	Presentation in Postmenopausal Women
Table 1 **(continued)**		
Nontumorous hyperandrogenisms *Iatrogenic causes*		
Medication use	Glucocorticoids	*Sx:* Stigmata of glucocorticoid excess *Data:* Elevated cortisol on laboratory tests, suppressed gonadotropins
	Androgens Antiepileptics	*Sx:* Rapid virilization temporally related to medication/ supplement start *Data:* Severe elevations in T and/or DHEAS; suppressed gonadotropins
Medication abuse	Anabolic steroids Pellets	*Sx:* Rapid virilization temporally related to medication/ supplement start *Data:* Severe elevations in T and/or DHEAS; suppressed gonadotropins
Tumorous hyperandrogenism *Adrenal causes*		
Adrenal adenomas		*Sx:* mild to moderate hyperandrogenism and hypercortisolism *Data:* Elevated T, usually with concurrent mild to moderate hypercortisolism; suppressed ACTH and DHEAS
Adrenal carcinomas		*Sx:* Rapid virilization often with stigmata of hypercortisolism *Data:* T $\geq$150 ng/dL, DHEAS >800 ng/mL, with cosecretion of other adrenal hormones, usually glucocorticoids; >8- to 10-cm mass seen on imaging
Tumorous hyperandrogenism *Ovarian causes*		
Sertoli-Leydig cell tumors		*Sx:* Rapid virilization *Data:* T 150 ng/dL; larger tumors (3–12 cm) at presentation, unilateral

(continued on next page)

Table 1 (continued)	
Diagnosis	Presentation in Postmenopausal Women
Granulosa cell tumors	Sx: Predominantly estrogen-secreting but 10% cosecrete androgens leading to rapid virilization; postmenopausal bleeding, endometrial hyperplasia, and endometrial carcinoma Data: T ≥150 ng/dL; larger tumors (3–12 cm) at presentation, cystic-appearing
Metastatic tumors cystadenomas	Sx: Rapid virilization; in metastatic tumors, signs of systemic illness Data: Paracrine action of β-hCG stimulates androgen secretion, stromal hyperplasia

Abbreviations: ACTH, adrenocorticotropic hormone; DST, dexamethasone suppression test; Sx, symptoms; UFC, urinary free cortisol; US, ultrasound.
    Data from Refs.[6,21,27]

androgen levels than women without PCOS.[7,12] Weight gain may also exacerbate hyperandrogenic symptoms in this population.[10,11] A careful menstrual history focusing on cycle regularity, timing of onset and progression of hyperandrogenic symptoms, and weight gain before menopause will help to elucidate this diagnosis.

Congenital Adrenal Hyperplasia

Like PCOS, congenital adrenal hyperplasia (CAH) is another potential cause of postmenopausal hyperandrogenism that typically presents before the menopausal transition. Both classical (rare) and nonclassical (more common) CAH should be on the differential for postmenopausal hyperandrogenism, particularly in individuals with a family history of early pubarche, short stature, and certain ethnic backgrounds.[13] However, it is important to note that screening for classical CAH owing to 21-hydroxylase deficiency is routinely done in newborns in the United States.

Obesity-Induced Hyperandrogenism

Nearly 40% of all postmenopausal women may be overweight/obese, but not all have PCOS.[14] A common presentation within the authors' clinical practice that has not been rigorously defined is "obesity-induced hyperandrogenism." Obesity-induced hyperandrogenism is distinguishable from PCOS, as these women usually have normal menstrual cyclicity throughout life, but have a history of progressive weight gain, often with successive pregnancies, without a return to baseline weight. At a certain weight threshold (differing for each individual), the menstrual cycle becomes irregular with development of hyperandrogenic signs. Development of hyperandrogenic symptoms is in part due to reduced levels of SHBG in obesity leading to increased circulating free androgens.[15] The authors further hypothesize that excess aromatase and 5-alpha-reductase in adipose tissue cause increased local estrogens and androgens that lead to irregular menses, hirsutism, and acne.[6] A similar cascade of events may also occur in postmenopausal women if their weight reaches the individual threshold after the menopausal transition. Therefore, a careful weight history focusing on the trajectory and timing of weight gain will help differentiate between PCOS and obesity-induced hyperandrogenism. Another clue is whether hyperandrogenic signs and symptoms might improve with weight loss, as the hyperandrogenic symptoms of obesity-induced hyperandrogenism may be more responsive to weight loss. Unfortunately, there are no head-to-head studies comparing changes in androgen levels in women with PCOS after menopause versus women with obesity with similar body mass index without a prior history of PCOS.

Hyperthecosis

A rare, nontumorous cause of hyperandrogenism is hyperthecosis, although this condition is often hard to differentiate from both PCOS and tumorous causes. In a 2018 study by Elhassan and colleagues,[16] hyperthecosis accounted for up to 9.3% of all cases of postmenopausal hyperandrogenism in 1205 consecutively recruited women. Obtaining a history of PCOS signs and symptoms is important, as hyperthecosis is considered a severe form of PCOS with considerable overlap in clinical manifestations and metabolic consequences.[17] Although the extent of symptoms with hyperthecosis can be as extreme as those with a tumor, they typically develop over several years, often beginning in the premenopausal period. The exact cause is unknown but results from the overproduction of androgens in the ovarian stromal cells and relates to elevated gonadotropins characteristic of menopause.[18,19] In addition, women with hyperthecosis have high degrees of insulin resistance that further drives production of ovarian androgens.[20] The ovarian volume in women with hyperthecosis generally exceeds 10 cm^3, which may be a normal ovarian size in premenopausal but not in postmenopausal women (where the typical volume is between 2.5 and 3.7 cm^3).[19] Therefore, it is important to consider both age and menopausal status when interpreting pelvic ultrasound findings. Serum levels of testosterone (>150 ng/dL) and estrogen are elevated, which may confer an increased risk of endometrial hyperplasia and carcinoma.[19,21] In addition, women with postmenopausal ovarian hyperthecosis are at risk for developing the metabolic syndrome, with conditions such as obesity, hypertension, hyperlipidemia, insulin resistance, hyperinsulinemia, and type 2 diabetes.[19,20,22] Ultimately, the diagnosis of hyperthecosis is made on histopathology.

Tumors of the Adrenal or Ovary

There may be considerable overlap in hyperandrogenic and virilizing symptoms between hyperthecosis and tumorous causes. However, severe postmenopausal hyperandrogenism that is rapid in onset generally points toward a neoplastic process. These women have evidence of virilization owing to high levels of circulating androgens. Old photographs may be helpful to review. Androgen-secreting tumors may be either adrenal or ovarian in origin.

Adrenal adenomas

Adrenal adenomas are the most common type of adrenal tumors, and they may be malignant or benign and secretory or nonfunctional.[23] Androgen-secreting tumors are ones that produce androgenic prohormones: dehydroepiandrostenedione (DHEA), dehydroepiandrostenedione sulfate (DHEAS), glucocorticoids, and/or estrogens; they rarely secrete testosterone.[24] A 2004 study by Moreno and colleagues[25] found that out of 801 consecutive adrenal operations from 1970 through 2003, only 21 patients had a pure androgen-secreting tumor. Adrenal carcinomas represent a rare cause of androgen-secreting adrenal tumors (annual incidence of 0.7–2 cases per million) and are more likely to lead to hyperandrogenism in postmenopausal women through cosecretion of DHEAS and glucocorticoids; secretion of androstenedione and testosterone is also common in postmenopausal women with adrenal carcinomas.[16,26,27] These tumors grow slowly and are typically diagnosed once they are larger than 8 to 10 cm.[28] In contrast, patients with adrenal Cushing syndrome may present with subtle hypercortisolism, elevated testosterone levels, but low DHEAS levels, as the tumor will shut off the normal hypothalamic-pituitary-adrenal axis.[29]

Ovarian androgen-secreting tumors

Ovarian androgen-secreting tumors arise from either the sex cord cells surrounding the oocyte (theca and granulosa cells) or from stromal cells. Sex cord–stromal tumors are rare and represent approximately 5% to 8% of all ovarian tumors. They are further divided based on their cell of origin and include Leydig cell tumors, Sertoli cell tumors, granulosa cell tumors, ovarian thecomas, and steroid cell tumors, not otherwise specified; less than half are androgen secreting. The Sertoli-Leydig tumors, for example, comprise 0.5% of all ovarian tumors and approximately one-fourth present after menopause.[21,27] Pure Leydig cell tumors secrete androgens, whereas pure Sertoli cells secrete estrogens. Both Sertoli and Leydig cell tumors are often relatively large in size, unilateral, and confined to the ovary at the time of diagnosis.[21] They are rarely malignant, although this depends on the degree of differentiation at diagnosis, but may exhibit early recurrence after resection.[30] Granulosa cell tumors similarly present at an early stage and exhibit good prognosis, although late recurrences and metastases requiring chemotherapy can occur. They account for 2% to 3% of all ovarian tumors and typically present in the sixth decade of life.[31] Granulosa cell tumors primarily secrete estrogens and lead to postmenopausal bleeding, endometrial hyperplasia, and endometrial carcinoma. However, up to 10% may secrete androgens leading to virilization.[31,32] Among epithelial tumors, serous cystadenomas are the most common, presenting in the fourth or fifth decade of life. Although not steroidogenic, they can secrete β-human chorionic gonadotropin (β-hCG), which can stimulate androgen secretion via paracrine action. Stromal hyperplasia can occur as a result.[21,27,33] Rarely, androgen secretion can occur from similar paracrine activity from metastases of neuroendocrine tumors to the ovaries.

Iatrogenic Hyperandrogenism

Medications and/or supplements may contribute to postmenopausal hyperandrogenism.[4] Most common are anabolic (eg, danazol) or androgenic steroids (eg, testosterone, DHEA, androstenedione) that may be used by athletes, included in dietary supplements, or used for low energy or sexual dysfunction.[27] Some clinicians are prescribing compounded combinations of estrogens with testosterone or DHEA for hypoactive sexual desire disorder. The Endocrine Society recommends against the routine diagnosis of androgen deficiency syndrome, as there are limited data correlating androgen levels with specific symptoms.[34] Although a high physiologic dose of testosterone in postmenopausal women has shown short-term efficacy and safety, the use of non–Food and Drug Administration–approved "bioidentical hormonal therapy" is thought to cause more harm than benefit.[35] The use of such therapies as pellets containing testosterone, estrogen, and progesterone, which are often promoted on the Internet or inserted at antiaging clinics, can cause serum testosterone levels to escalate into the male range, leading to rapid onset of acne, virilization, mood changes, male pattern balding, and hyperlipidemia. Furthermore, it may take many months for testosterone levels to return to the normal postmenopausal range after discontinuation.[36] Exposure to a partner's testosterone gel may lead to milder symptoms of androgen excess. Antiepileptics, such as valproic acid, or glucocorticoids may be additional iatrogenic causes of hyperandrogenism. A careful review of all medications, supplements, and partner's hormonal therapies is key in detecting these reversible causes of postmenopausal hyperandrogenism.

Endocrinopathies

The major endocrinopathies to consider in postmenopausal women that may lead to androgen excess are Cushing syndrome, hyperprolactinemia, and acromegaly. Half of the patients with Cushing syndrome may have hirsutism from adrenal androgen excess; hypercortisolism also correlates with increased free androgens, likely because of decreased SHBG.[21,37] As previously discussed, androgens may also be cosecreted with cortisol in adrenal carcinomas. In contrast, women with adrenocorticotropin-dependent Cushing disease have mild hirsutism. Hyperprolactinemia from medications or thyroid disorders also can cause hirsutism in premenopausal women that has been shown to improve with dopamine agonist therapy, suggesting that prolactin may lead to increased adrenal androgen production.[38,39] Because high estrogen levels can stimulate prolactin secretion, elevated prolactin levels and associated symptoms may improve after menopause.[40]

Acromegaly is a rare cause of postmenopausal hyperandrogenism, although up to 50% of women with growth hormone (GH) excess can have hirsutism.[41] In premenopausal women with acromegaly, GH hypersecretion leads to increased insulin-like growth factor-1 (IGF-1) levels along with hyperinsulinemia that stimulates ovarian androgen production.[41,42] There are also several, rarer endocrinopathies, such as glucocorticoid-resistant states, altered glucocorticoid metabolism, and androgen insensitivity states, that can present in postmenopausal women, but these are typically diagnosed earlier in life.[21] It is important to keep the list of endocrinopathies in the differential framework for postmenopausal hyperandrogenism, as it will impact the diagnostic workup.

DIAGNOSTIC EVALUATION

The history and physical examination help direct appropriate steps in laboratory and radiologic evaluation (outlined in **Fig. 1**). It is useful to start with laboratory evaluation to help select imaging modality, particularly with suspected adrenal causes, because an adrenal adenoma can be detected in up to 7% of the elderly population.[29]

Laboratory Testing

The most important androgens to check are total testosterone level and DHEAS, although androstenedione may be a useful prohormone to measure. The normal concentrations of these androgens in postmenopausal women vary by age and laboratory normal ranges. Measuring DHEA is not recommended, as it is a pulsatile hormone. Most commercial total testosterone assays are radioimmunoassays developed for testing levels in men and are frequently insensitive for detection of lower levels of testosterone in women.[43] Liquid chromatography–tandem mass spectrometry is considered the gold standard for measuring total testosterone level in women given its high sensitivity and specificity.[44] Free testosterone measured by direct assays are generally unreliable but can be useful if measured by equilibrium dialysis.[43] Hyperandrogenism in postmenopausal women should be interpreted in the context that both adrenal and ovarian androgens decline with age in women.[45]

There are some general guidelines on distinguishing tumorous and nontumorous causes of androgen excess on laboratory tests. For example, a total testosterone

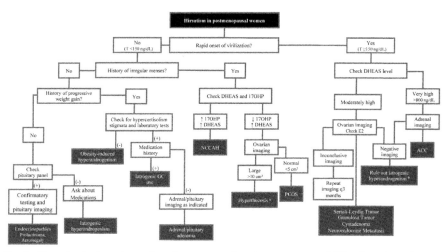

Fig. 1. Flowchart of workup of postmenopausal androgen excess. ACC, adrenal carcinoma; GC, glucocorticoid; E2, estradiol; NCCAH, nonclassical congenital adrenal hyperplasia; T, testosterone. [a] In many cases of hyperthecosis, T may be $\geq$150 ng/dL. [b] If negative for iatrogenic hyperandrogenism, consider performing ovarian-adrenal vein sampling. (*Data from* Refs.[6,21,27])

level less than 150 ng/dL (5.2 nmol/L) generally indicates a nontumorous cause, especially when virilization is not present. However, no threshold definitively separates benign from malignant processes.[21,46] It can be difficult to differentiate hyperthecosis from ovarian tumors on laboratory evaluation alone.[47] Although a retrospective study of 34 patients showed that postmenopausal women with ovarian tumors had higher testosterone/estradiol levels and lower gonadotropins compared with women with hyperthecosis, there was a great deal of overlap in hormonal profiles between the 2 conditions.[18] Both groups had total testosterone levels greater than 150 ng/dL, although levels in women with ovarian tumors were nearly 3-fold higher (560 $\pm$ 434 ng/dL in tumors vs 182 $\pm$ 89 ng/dL in hyperthecosis). The gonadotropin-releasing hormone (GnRH) analogue suppression test has been used to determine if testosterone excess originates from the ovaries; however, its utility in distinguishing hyperthecosis from an ovarian tumor is limited. In small studies of women with hyperthecosis or ovarian tumors, the GnRH suppression test resulted in suppression of gonadotropins as well as a reduction in testosterone levels by at least 50% in both groups.[18,48] Historically, a DHEAS level greater than 800 ng/mL (2171 nmol/L) with a total testosterone level greater than 200 ng/dL (6.94 nmol/L) pointed toward a tumorous cause.[6] In Elhassan's 2018 study, severe DHEAS elevations were found exclusively in adrenal carcinoma.[16] Interestingly, very high DHEAS in premenopausal women was predominantly due to PCOS. Severe androstenedione excess was also a marker of adrenal carcinoma in postmenopausal women, whereas mild elevations in androstenedione were more likely related to PCOS.

Other laboratory tests should be obtained based on clinical suspicion from the history and physical examination. These tests primarily include ruling out CAH or the list of endocrinopathies. A prolactin level can be obtained in the setting of associated galactorrhea or medications that may cause hyperprolactinemia. A borderline 17-hydroxyprogesterone (17OHP) level should be followed by testing 30 minutes after intravenous cosyntropin to rule out CAH.[13] Cushing syndrome should also be excluded with 2 of the 3 of the following tests: 24-hour urinary free cortisol, 1-mg overnight dexamethasone suppression test, and salivary free cortisol.[23,49] If there is suspicion of acromegaly, an IGF-1 level should be drawn, and if elevated, confirmation testing can be performed with an oral glucose tolerance test.[50] Based on laboratory findings, specific imaging modalities can be used for localization of potential causes.

Radiologic Evaluation

When history/physical examination and laboratory evaluation point to an adrenal or ovarian cause of androgen excess, imaging studies should be the next step. Ovarian tumors are often small but can be identified using transvaginal ultrasonography (TVUS) or MRI. In a study of 22 postmenopausal women with both tumorous and nontumorous causes of androgen excess, MRI was found to be more sensitive and specific with higher positive predictive (78%) and negative predictive (100%) values versus TVUS in detecting ovarian tumors.[21,46] In cases whereby a clear ovarian tumor cannot be identified, asymmetry of the ovaries may suggest a lesion, and imaging should be repeated at 3-month intervals.[6]

As previously mentioned, adrenal tumors that cause hyperandrogenism are typically greater than 8 to 10 cm at the time of presentation. However, computed axial tomography (CT) or MRI of the adrenals is indicated in a hyperandrogenic woman with a high DHEAS and other clinical concerns for Cushing syndrome. Measuring Hounsfield units (HU) in a noncontrast CT scan can help distinguish adrenal carcinomas from benign adenomas. Low fat content (high density; >10 HU) correlates with malignancy with a sensitivity and specificity close to 71% and 98%, respectively. On a CT scan with delayed contrast media washout, a 50% washout and absolute value of 35 HU after 10 to 15 minutes have superior diagnostic accuracy. With MRI, adrenal carcinomas appear heterogenous, often with necrosis or calcification, and bright because of their high water content.[26,27] A pituitary MRI with and without contrast is indicated when history and data point to endocrinopathies, such as acromegaly or hyperprolactinemia.

If TVUS, CT, and MRI are unable to localize the androgen-secreting tumor, combined ovarian and adrenal vein sampling can be considered. However, the data do not support its ability to reliably change management. The ovary is likely to be the source in these cases given their small size at diagnosis. The process is tedious and requires catheterization of all 4 veins (right/left adrenal and right/left ovarian) to detect a left-to-right difference in androgen concentrations.[3,51] In a series of 38 patients from St Bartholomew's Hospital in London, successful catheterization of all 4 veins was only 27%. In 2 of the 38 patients whereby vein sampling indicated a tumor, the final pathology was consistent with PCOS. Adrenal and ovarian vein sampling is not widely performed and should be considered only in centers with expertise.[51]

TREATMENT BENEFITS AND OPTIONS

Treatments to reduce androgen levels may be important for metabolic and cardiovascular concerns as well as for quality of life. However, the degree to which elevated androgens confer risk of cardiovascular disease (CVD) has been debated. Although women with PCOS often have accompanying insulin resistance and obesity along with dyslipidemia and hyperandrogenism, increased cardiovascular risk has not been well established in this population.[52,53] In studies of transgender men, who have been exposed to androgens long term, excess risk for CVD has not been consistently demonstrated.[54] However, much of these data is in younger patients where cardiovascular risk is generally low, and longer-term prospective studies are needed. In postmenopausal women with virilizing tumors and very high androgen levels, hypertension and dyslipidemia have been reported, but it remains unclear whether these abnormalities increase CVD risk and how effectively tumor removal will optimize metabolic alterations.[55] Nonetheless, treatment is frequently used to remove the inciting cause and improve patient distress related to androgenic symptoms.

Treatment strategies depend on the cause of androgen excess. Tumorous causes generally require surgical resection. Although the diagnosis of hyperthecosis is ultimately made by histopathology, many of the sequelae in this condition are driven by insulin resistance. Lifestyle changes, weight loss, and insulin sensitizers can improve testosterone to normal postmenopausal levels,[17,47,56] but more commonly, bilateral oophorectomy is indicated. GnRH analogues can be used as a medical castration to treat hyperthecosis or ovarian tumors if the patient is not a surgical candidate or if a tumor is not identified on imaging.[19,20,57] Insulin sensitizers can suppress androgens in premenopausal women with PCOS,[58] although data in postmenopausal women are lacking. Postmenopausal women with nonclassical CAH may be treated similarly to PCOS patients, although the addition of hydrocortisone may sometimes be indicated, similar to classical CAH patients.[13] Iatrogenic causes of hyperandrogenism can be ameliorated by discontinuation of the causative medication/supplement. Hyperandrogenism from endocrinopathies should be approached using the diagnostic and treatment guidelines for the specific condition. Finally, treatment can also target symptom reduction. For example, hirsutism may be ameliorated with antiandrogens, such as spironolactone or flutamide. Cyproterone acetate can also be used, although it is not available in the United States.[4]

SUMMARY

Evidence of clinical and/or biochemical androgen excess poses a unique differential in postmenopausal women. Some signs and symptoms of postmenopausal hyperandrogenism can be normal and attributed to the natural aging process. However, the causes of androgen excess in this group include both nontumorous and tumorous causes. Treatment of androgen excess in postmenopausal women may improve both quality of life and long-term metabolic outcomes.

CLINICS CARE POINTS

- Symptoms of mild postmenopausal hyperandrogenism are common; however, a workup is often indicated to assess the cause.
- The development of rapid and true virilizing signs signals a need to quickly assess for malignancy.
- A focused history and physical examination with appropriate laboratory and radiologic evaluation can differentiate tumorous from nontumorous causes of postmenopausal hyperandrogenism, leading to optimal treatment strategies.

DISCLOSURE

Dr A. Zaman has received grant F32 DK123878 from NIH. The other author has nothing to disclose.

REFERENCES

1. Fogle RH, Stanczyk FZ, Zhang X, et al. Ovarian androgen production in postmenopausal women. J Clin Endocrinol Metab 2007;92(8):3040–3.
2. Gershagen S, Doeberl A, Jeppsson S, et al. Decreasing serum levels of sex hormone-binding globulin around the menopause and temporary relation to changing levels of ovarian steroids, as demonstrated in a longitudinal study. Fertil Steril 1989;51(4):616–21.
3. Alpanes M, Gonzalez-Casbas JM, Sanchez J, et al. Management of postmenopausal virilization. J Clin Endocrinol Metab 2012;97(8):2584–8.
4. Martin KA, Anderson RR, Chang RJ, et al. Evaluation and treatment of hirsutism in premenopausal women: an Endocrine Society Clinical Practice Guideline. J Clin Endocrinol Metab 2018;103(4):1233–57.
5. Ferriman D, Gallwey JD. Clinical assessment of body hair growth in women. J Clin Endocrinol Metab 1961;21:1440–7.
6. Rothman MS, Wierman ME. How should postmenopausal androgen excess be evaluated? Clin Endocrinol (Oxf) 2011;75(2):160–4.
7. Azziz R, Carmina E, Chen Z, et al. Polycystic ovary syndrome. Nat Rev Dis Primers 2016;2:16057.
8. Bozdag G, Mumusoglu S, Zengin D, et al. The prevalence and phenotypic features of polycystic ovary syndrome: a systematic review and meta-analysis. Hum Reprod 2016;31(12):2841–55.
9. Azziz R, Carmina E, Dewailly D, et al. The Androgen Excess and PCOS Society criteria for the polycystic ovary syndrome: the complete task force report. Fertil Steril 2009;91(2):456–88.
10. Rotterdam EA-SPCWG. Revised 2003 consensus on diagnostic criteria and long-term health risks related to polycystic ovary syndrome. Fertil Steril 2004;81(1):19–25.
11. Legro RS, Arslanian SA, Ehrmann DA, et al. Diagnosis and treatment of polycystic ovary syndrome: an Endocrine Society Clinical Practice Guideline. J Clin Endocrinol Metab 2013;98(12):4565–92.
12. Markopoulos MC, Rizos D, Valsamakis G, et al. Hyperandrogenism in women with polycystic ovary syndrome persists after menopause. J Clin Endocrinol Metab 2011;96(3):623–31.
13. Speiser PW, Arlt W, Auchus RJ, et al. Congenital adrenal hyperplasia due to steroid 21-hydroxylase deficiency: an Endocrine Society Clinical Practice Guideline. J Clin Endocrinol Metab 2018;103(11):4043–88.
14. Hales CM, Fryar CD, Carroll MD, et al. Trends in obesity and severe obesity prevalence in US youth and adults by sex and age, 2007-2008 to 2015-2016. JAMA 2018;319(16):1723–5.
15. Pasquali R. Obesity and androgens: facts and perspectives. Fertil Steril 2006;85(5):1319–40.
16. Elhassan YS, Idkowiak J, Smith K, et al. Causes, patterns, and severity of androgen excess in 1205 consecutively recruited women. J Clin Endocrinol Metab 2018;103(3):1214–23.
17. Vaikkakara S, Al-Ozairi E, Lim E, et al. The investigation and management of severe hyperandrogenism pre- and postmenopause: non-tumor disease is strongly associated with metabolic syndrome and typically responds to insulin-sensitization with metformin. Gynecol Endocrinol 2008;24(2):87–92.

18. Yance VRV, Marcondes JAM, Rocha MP, et al. Discriminating between virilizing ovary tumors and ovary hyperthecosis in postmenopausal women: clinical data, hormonal profiles and image studies. Eur J Endocrinol 2017;177(1):93–102.
19. Krug E, Berga SL. Postmenopausal hyperthecosis: functional dysregulation of androgenesis in climacteric ovary. Obstet Gynecol 2002;99(5 Pt 2):893–7.
20. Barth JH, Jenkins M, Belchetz PE. Ovarian hyperthecosis, diabetes and hirsuties in post-menopausal women. Clin Endocrinol (Oxf) 1997;46(2):123–8.
21. Markopoulos MC, Kassi E, Alexandraki KI, et al. Hyperandrogenism after menopause. Eur J Endocrinol 2015;172(2):R79–91.
22. Rittmaster RS. Polycystic ovary syndrome, hyperthecosis and the menopause. Clin Endocrinol (Oxf) 1997;46(2):129–30.
23. Nieman LK. Approach to the patient with an adrenal incidentaloma. J Clin Endocrinol Metab 2010;95(9):4106–13.
24. Zhou WB, Chen N, Li CJ. A rare case of pure testosterone-secreting adrenal adenoma in a postmenopausal elderly woman. BMC Endocr Disord 2019;19(1):14.
25. Moreno S, Montoya G, Armstrong J, et al. Profile and outcome of pure androgen-secreting adrenal tumors in women: experience of 21 cases. Surgery 2004; 136(6):1192–8.
26. Kassi E, Angelousi A, Zografos G, et al. Current issues in the diagnosis and management of adrenocortical carcinomas. [Updated 2016 Mar 6]. In: Feingold KR, Anawalt B, Boyce A, et al, editors. Endotext [Internet]. South Dartmouth (MA): MDText.com, Inc.; 2000. Available at: https://www.ncbi.nlm.nih.gov/books/NBK279009/.
27. Ervin K, Kostakis LNG, Macut D, et al. Androgens in menopausal women: not only polycystic ovary syndrome. In: Renato Pasquali DP, editor. Hyperandrogenism in women: beyond polycystic ovary syndrome, vol. 53. Basel: Karger; 2019. p. 135–61.
28. Cordera F, Grant C, van Heerden J, et al. Androgen-secreting adrenal tumors. Surgery 2003;134(6):874–80 [discussion: 880].
29. Young WF Jr. Clinical practice. The incidentally discovered adrenal mass. N Engl J Med 2007;356(6):601–10.
30. Gui T, Cao D, Shen K, et al. A clinicopathological analysis of 40 cases of ovarian Sertoli-Leydig cell tumors. Gynecol Oncol 2012;127(2):384–9.
31. Sekkate S, Kairouani M, Serji B, et al. Ovarian granulosa cell tumors: a retrospective study of 27 cases and a review of the literature. World J Surg Oncol 2013; 11:142.
32. Nakashima N, Young RH, Scully RE. Androgenic granulosa cell tumors of the ovary. A clinicopathologic analysis of 17 cases and review of the literature. Arch Pathol Lab Med 1984;108(10):786–91.
33. Heinonen PK, Morsky P, Aine R, et al. Hormonal activity of epithelial ovarian tumours in post-menopausal women. Maturitas 1988;9(4):325–38.
34. Wierman ME, Arlt W, Basson R, et al. Androgen therapy in women: a reappraisal: an Endocrine Society Clinical Practice Guideline. J Clin Endocrinol Metab 2014; 99(10):3489–510.
35. Santoro N, Braunstein GD, Butts CL, et al. Compounded bioidentical hormones in endocrinology practice: an Endocrine Society Scientific Statement. J Clin Endocrinol Metab 2016;101(4):1318–43.
36. Seaborg E. Targeting patients with pellets: a look at bioidentical hormones. In: Newman MA, Bagley D, editors. Endocrine News. Washington, DC: Endocrine Society; 2019. p. 22–7.

37. Kaltsas GA, Korbonits M, Isidori AM, et al. How common are polycystic ovaries and the polycystic ovarian syndrome in women with Cushing's syndrome? Clin Endocrinol (Oxf) 2000;53(4):493–500.

38. Tirgar-Tabari S, Sharbatdaran M, Manafi-Afkham S, et al. Hyperprolactinemia and hirsutism in patients without polycystic ovary syndrome. Int J Trichology 2016; 8(3):130–4.

39. Hagag P, Hertzianu I, Ben-Shlomo A, et al. Androgen suppression and clinical improvement with dopamine agonists in hyperandrogenic-hyperprolactinemic women. J Reprod Med 2001;46(7):678–84.

40. Faje AT, Klibanski A. The treatment of hyperprolactinemia in postmenopausal women with prolactin-secreting microadenomas: cons. Endocrine 2015;48(1): 79–82.

41. Kaltsas GA, Mukherjee JJ, Jenkins PJ, et al. Menstrual irregularity in women with acromegaly. J Clin Endocrinol Metab 1999;84(8):2731–5.

42. Kaltsas GA, Androulakis II, Tziveriotis K, et al. Polycystic ovaries and the polycystic ovary syndrome phenotype in women with active acromegaly. Clin Endocrinol (Oxf) 2007;67(6):917–22.

43. Rosner W, Auchus RJ, Azziz R, et al. Position statement: utility, limitations, and pitfalls in measuring testosterone: an Endocrine Society position statement. J Clin Endocrinol Metab 2007;92(2):405–13.

44. Pugeat M, Plotton I, de la Perriere AB, et al. Management of endocrine disease hyperandrogenic states in women: pitfalls in laboratory diagnosis. Eur J Endocrinol 2018;178(4):R141–54.

45. Davison SL, Bell R, Donath S, et al. Androgen levels in adult females: changes with age, menopause, and oophorectomy. J Clin Endocrinol Metab 2005;90(7): 3847–53.

46. Sarfati J, Bachelot A, Coussieu C, Meduri G, Touraine P, Study Group Hyperandrogenism in Postmenopausal Women. Impact of clinical, hormonal, radiological, and immunohistochemical studies on the diagnosis of postmenopausal hyperandrogenism. Eur J Endocrinol 2011;165(5):779–88.

47. Mamoojee Y, Ganguri M, Taylor N, et al. Clinical case seminar: postmenopausal androgen excess-challenges in diagnostic work-up and management of ovarian thecosis. Clin Endocrinol (Oxf) 2018;88(1):13–20.

48. Pascale MM, Pugeat M, Roberts M, et al. Androgen suppressive effect of GnRH agonist in ovarian hyperthecosis and virilizing tumours. Clin Endocrinol (Oxf) 1994;41(5):571–6.

49. Thompson GB, Young WF Jr. Adrenal incidentaloma. Curr Opin Oncol 2003; 15(1):84–90.

50. Katznelson L, Laws ER Jr, Melmed S, et al. Acromegaly: an Endocrine Society Clinical Practice Guideline. J Clin Endocrinol Metab 2014;99(11):3933–51.

51. Kaltsas GA, Mukherjee JJ, Kola B, et al. Is ovarian and adrenal venous catheterization and sampling helpful in the investigation of hyperandrogenic women? Clin Endocrinol (Oxf) 2003;59(1):34–43.

52. Torchen LC. Cardiometabolic risk in PCOS: more than a reproductive disorder. Curr Diab Rep 2017;17(12):137.

53. Anagnostis P, Tarlatzis BC, Kauffman RP. Polycystic ovarian syndrome (PCOS): long-term metabolic consequences. Metabolism 2018;86:33–43.

54. Irwig MS. Cardiovascular health in transgender people. Rev Endocr Metab Disord 2018;19(3):243–51.

55. Rocha T, Crespo RP, Yance VVR, et al. Persistent poor metabolic profile in post-menopausal women with ovarian hyperandrogenism after testosterone level normalization. J Endocr Soc 2019;3(5):1087–96.
56. Al-Ozairi E, Michael E, Quinton R. Insulin resistance causing severe postmeno-pausal hyperandrogenism. Int J Gynaecol Obstet 2008;100(3):280–1.
57. Vollaard ES, van Beek AP, Verburg FA, et al. Gonadotropin-releasing hormone agonist treatment in postmenopausal women with hyperandrogenism of ovarian origin. J Clin Endocrinol Metab 2011;96(5):1197–201.
58. Katsiki N, Hatzitolios AI. Insulin-sensitizing agents in the treatment of polycystic ovary syndrome: an update. Curr Opin Obstet Gynecol 2010;22(6):466–76.

Use of Testosterone in Postmenopausal Women

Susan R. Davis, MBBS, FRACP, PhD, FAHMS

KEYWORDS

- Testosterone therapy • Postmenopausal women • Female sexual dysfunction

KEY POINTS

- The only evidence-based indication for testosterone supplementation in women is for the treatment of postmenopausal women with low sexual desire with associated personal distress.
- Based on the available data, testosterone supplementation should not be used to improve cardiometabolic, musculoskeletal, or cognitive health; well-being and low mood; or vasomotor symptoms in postmenopausal women; there currently are insufficient data to support the use of testosterone in premenopausal women.
- The use of compounded testosterone formulations is discouraged, and, when these are the only treatment options, adherence to the highest manufacturing standard is required.
- Testosterone supplementation for women with hypoactive sexual desire disorder always should be considered a trial of therapy.

INTRODUCTION

Testosterone is an important sex steroid in women that can act directly as an androgen or be aromatized to estradiol (E_2) in target tissues, resulting in with pleiotropic effects.[1] Because testosterone is an obligatory precursor for estrogen production, it has been difficult to differentiate the independent effects of testosterone from estrogen for some clinical outcomes. Currently, in terms of testosterone supplementation, the only accepted evidenced-based indication is for the treatment of low sexual desire with associated with personal distress (hypoactive sexual desire disorder [HSDD]) in postmenopausal women.[2] Although in vitro and observational studies suggest low endogenous testosterone in postmenopausal women may be associated with a greater risk of both cardiovascular (CV) disease and fragility fracture,[3] no large, well-powered, randomized controlled trial (RCT) has evaluated these effects as primary outcomes. With respect to testosterone supplementation, the recommendations are that nonoral therapy should be used, because this is not associated with adverse lipid effects seen with oral testosterone, and that the prescribed dose should result in

Women's Health Research Program, School of Public Health and Preventive Medicine, Monash University, 553 St Kilda Road, Melbourne, Victoria 3004, Australia
E-mail address: susan.davis@monash.edu

Endocrinol Metab Clin N Am 50 (2021) 113–124
https://doi.org/10.1016/j.ecl.2020.11.002
0889-8529/21/© 2020 Elsevier Inc. All rights reserved.
endo.theclinics.com

physiologic blood testosterone concentrations that approximate those of premenopausal women.[2]

OVERVIEW OF THE PHYSIOLOGY OF TESTOSTERONE IN WOMEN

In healthy, regularly menstruating premenopausal women, median serum testosterone concentrations, measured by liquid chromatography–tandem mass spectrometry (LC-MS/MS), are similar to those of E_2 (300–400 pmol/L or 82–109 pg/mL).[4] In premenopausal women, however, testosterone levels decline by approximately 25% between the third and fifth decades of life, so that by the time women reach the average age of natural menopause their testosterone levels are substantially lower than when they were younger.

In postmenopausal women, testosterone is made primarily in peripheral tissues from its circulating, less active, adrenal precursors, dehydroepiandrosterone and androstenedione. Within the cells in which it is produced, testosterone may be metabolized further to the more potent androgen, dihydrotestosterone, or aromatized to E_2, which then acts locally. Therefore, testosterone exerts its actions directly as an androgen or indirectly as an estrogen precursor in women. The amount of testosterone produced after menopause is dependent on both the availability of the adrenal precursors (reflecting adrenal function) and the activity of the enzymes important in testosterone biosynthesis at the cellular level. Consequently, there are considerable variations in blood concentrations between women, and there is no blood concentration of testosterone below which a woman can be diagnosed as having testosterone deficiency.

Testosterone circulates mostly strongly bound to sex hormone–binding globulin (SHBG) (approximately 66%) and weakly bound to albumin (approximately 33%), with some weak binding to other plasma proteins.[5] It is widely assumed that non–protein-bound (free) testosterone (approximately 1%–2% of serum testosterone in women) is the biologically active component. Yet evidence that the free testosterone fraction is the biologically active fraction is lacking. It is equally likely that free testosterone is the most readily degradable fraction and, therefore, the least metabolically active component of circulating testosterone.[6] Furthermore, methods for measuring free testosterone are fraught with problems of poor precision and low specificity.[7] The different formulae commonly used to estimate free testosterone lack validity, in part because they assume linearity of binding of testosterone to SHBG, at all concentrations of each analyte, and hence the different formulae generate inconsistent results.[7] Until recently, measurement of total testosterone also was compromised by the insensitivity and poor precision of immunoassays at the low circulating testosterone concentrations in women, relative to men.[8] The increased availability of LC-MS/MS has made it possible to measure testosterone with precision in women.

Further complicating the picture, there is substantial evidence that SHBG, the protein that predominantly binds testosterone, also is metabolically active. SHBG levels vary substantially in women, with endogenous levels inversely linked to central adiposity and insulin levels.[9–11] SHBG is a strong independent marker of insulin resistance and type 2 diabetes mellitus risk[12] and has been implicated in the pathogenesis of type 2 diabetes mellitus and CV disease.[12] Strong, inverse relationships between both insulin resistance and SHBG, and between body mass index and SHBG,[13] independent of sex steroids have been demonstrated. Several studies evaluating testosterone action commonly estimate the free androgen index (FAI) (total testosterone/ SHBG × 100). In many studies, the FAI, but not total testosterone, has been associated with an adverse outcome.[14,15] Because the only factors in the calculation of the FAI are SHGB and testosterone, it can only be concluded SHBG is driving the associations reported, when total testosterone is unrelated to the outcome. Finally, studies investigating associations between endogenous testosterone levels and health outcomes are confounded by the biosynthesis and metabolism of testosterone in extragonadal tissues, such that circulating blood concentrations in women may not reflect tissue concentrations or tissue effects accurately.[16]

CURRENT EVIDENCE
Testosterone and Sexual Function

There are consistent signals that testosterone and its precursors are associated with self-reported sexual function in premenopausal[17–19] and postmenopausal women,[18,20] but the variation in sexual function explained by serum androgen concentrations in women is small.[19] Rather, sexual function/sexual well-being is determined predominantly by a range of other biopsychosocial factors.[21] For example, for premenopausal women, being partnered increases the likelihood of HSDD,[22] which increases to a 3-fold increase in risk for women at midlife.[23] Quality evidence that testosterone improves sexual function in postmenopausal women is limited to RCTs of postmenopausal women with HSDD.[24] A comprehensive systematic review and meta-analysis has reported that testosterone therapy results in statistically significant improvements in sexual desire, arousal, pleasure, orgasm frequency, and responsiveness; reduced sexual concerns in women assessed as having HSDD; and improved desire in women with generalized female sexual dysfunction (FSD). The Global Consensus Position Statement on the use of Testosterone Therapy for Women, published in 2019, concluded that the beneficial effects of testosterone therapy seen in women with HSDD or generalized FSD cannot be extrapolated to other subtypes of FSD or women without sexual dysfunction.[2]

The beneficial effects of testosterone on sexual functioning may involve both central and peripheral mechanisms. Testosterone replacement increases activation of brain areas associated with sexual function in estrogen-replete oophorectomized women.[25] In addition, testosterone may enhance arousal and orgasm by direct genital effects mediated by effects on vaginal androgen receptors (ARs) and enhancement of vasodilation.[26] Testosterone therapy increases vaginal AR gene expression,[26] increases vaginal blood flow,[27] and induces proliferation of vaginal epithelial cells in postmenopausal women.[28] These findings have led to the exploration of intravaginal testosterone as a potential treatment of vulvovaginal atrophy in women in general and in women taking aromatase inhibitor therapy after breast cancer.[29] Studies suggesting that intravaginal testosterone restores low vaginal pH, improves the vaginal maturation index, and enhances sexual function are limited mostly by lack of a placebo control,[30–32] short treatment duration,[30,31] nonadjustment for baseline differences,[33] and supraphysiologic testosterone dosing.[34] A small placebo-controlled RCT reported a 300-μg dose of testosterone applied intravaginally, 3 times per week for 26 weeks, significantly improved sexual satisfaction and responsiveness and reduced self-reported vaginal dryness, dyspareunia, sexual concerns, and sexually associated personal distress in women with breast cancer taking aromatase inhibitor therapy.[35] No improvement in the vaginal maturation index was demonstrated in this study. These findings require verification in a larger study.

Prevalence of Hypoactive Sexual Desire Disorder

Studies of the prevalence of low sexual desire and HSDD in women have yielded different findings, according to the nature of the participants (representative/convenience sample, nationality, partner status, and inclusion/exclusion of sexually inactive women), questionnaires used, and data collection methods (interview, face-to-face, or online questionnaire). The impact on estimated prevalences, according to who is included in the assessment of prevalence, is illustrated by contrasting findings reported by the British National Survey of Sexual Attitudes and Lifestyles (Natsal) and a large Australian study of a representative sample of older women that reported on sexual desire. Natsal-3 reported on sexual desire only for women with at least 1 sexual partner in the prior year.[36] The proportion of women aged 65 years to 74 years in Natsal-3 with low desire was 34.2%, compared, with more than 87% of women of this age in the Australian study.[36] Whereas Natsal-3 required women to be sexually active, in the Australian sample (which was representative of women of this age in the community), only 28% of the women aged 65 years to 74 years had been recently sexually active, accounting for the different prevalence estimates. These findings also fit with low desire being associated with avoidance of sexual activity.[37,38] Overall, most studies have found low sexual desire to become more prevalent with increasing age.[36,39–41]

Few studies have provided prevalence data for HSDD. The Prevalence of Female Sexual Problems Associated with Distress and Determinants of Treatment Seeking (PRESIDE) study, a large population-based survey of adult US women, reported a prevalence of HSDD of 12.4% for women aged 45 years to 64 years and 7.4% for women aged 65 years and older.[40] Two large Australian studies have reported prevalences of HSDD for women aged 40 years to 64 years and 65 years to 79 years to be 32.4% and 13.65%, respectively.[23,42] The different findings between the US and Australian studies may be due to the different sampling approaches and questionnaires or true sociocultural differences. In addition, the Australian surveys were conducted over 10 years after PRESIDE, so, potentially, with the increased public discussion about sexual function, women may have become more comfortable disclosing their sexual concerns. Notable in the Australian studies was that being partnered was associated with a 3-fold greater likelihood of HSDD in midlife women and 4-fold greater likelihood in older women.[23,42]

Testosterone and Other Health Outcomes

Despite the dogma that higher blood testosterone concentrations increase the risk of CV disease in women, in their review, Spoletini and colleagues[43] concluded that "a hypoandrogenic state [in women] is detrimental to cardiovascular (CV) health." This is because testosterone has been found to exert direct favorable vascular effects, including enhanced vasomotor tone and reduced peripheral vascular resistance.[44] Studies of postmenopausal women have shown increased endothelium-dependent (flow-mediated) and endothelium-independent brachial artery vasodilation.[45,46] These effects have been shown to not require aromatization of testosterone to E_2.[47] When acutely administered to postmenopausal women, testosterone is a vasodilator causing a mean drop in systolic blood pressure in the order of 10 mm Hg.[48] Testosterone has been shown to enhance cardiac muscle repolarization,[49] and it has been suggested that lower testosterone is associated with a greater risk of heart failure.[50]

Whereas no association between serum testosterone and CV disease is seen in younger women,[51] lower testosterone was associated with all-cause mortality and CV events in a study of 2914 women, mean age 58 years, with 4.5 years of follow-up.[52] An inverse association between serum testosterone and CV events has been reported by several other studies in postmenopausal women.[3] The findings need to be considered inconclusive, however, because studies have been limited by recruitment of convenience, clinic-based samples, case-control design, and long intervals between the time of blood draw and events. A majority also have used immunoassays, which lack the precision of LC-MS/MS, to measure testosterone. Studies suggesting an adverse effect of high testosterone on CV health also have reported on events decades after blood was drawn.[53,54] Only 1 small RCT has evaluated the impact of testosterone in women with CV disease. This placebo-controlled study reported improvement in exercise capacity and muscle strength in women with advanced heart failure.[55] Clearly more research into the role of testosterone levels and CV function is needed.

From a contemporary therapeutic perspective, there is no evidence that testosterone therapy, when used for the treatment of HSDD, is associated with adverse CV effects.[24]

Testosterone exerts anabolic actions in musculoskeletal tissue, mediated directly through ARs and indirectly by aromatization to E_2.[56] In postmenopausal women, higher free testosterone has been associated with higher bone density.[57] Higher SHBG and low free testosterone, however, but not total testosterone have been associated with a greater fracture risk.[58] In a longitudinal study of Japanese women, sarcopenia was associated with lower free testosterone but, again, not total testosterone.[59] These observations again indicate SHBG may have direct physiologic actions that need to be better understood. Interventional studies of testosterone that have evaluated musculoskeletal outcomes have provided inconclusive results.[24] These are due to small size, inconsistent reporting of outcome measures, and short treatment durations. Based on the available data, testosterone should not be used to prevent or treat bone loss or sarcopenia in postmenopausal women.

In vitro and in vivo studies have demonstrated neuroprotective and anti-inflammatory effects of testosterone in the central nervous system,[60] and small observational studies have reported higher endogenous testosterone associated with superior verbal fluency[61] and verbal memory performance in postmenopausal women.[62] In a clinical trial, in which postmenopausal women on transdermal E_2 also all were treated with transdermal testosterone, and then in a double-blind design, randomly allocated to letrozole or placebo, testosterone was associated with improved cognitive performance in both the letrozole and placebo groups.[63] This suggests that testosterone may exert favorable cognitive effects without requiring conversion to E_2. Subsequently, a small, 6-month double-blind RCT of transdermal testosterone, versus placebo, in postmenopausal women, aged 55 years to 65 years, not taking concurrent estrogen, found statistically significant improvements in verbal learning and memory, after adjustment for age and baseline scores.[64] Although these findings are provocative, a systematic review and meta-analysis of RCTs of testosterone with cognitive performance outcomes in postmenopausal women found no overall effect of testosterone on a range of cognitive measures.[24] Whether testosterone is protective against mild cognitive impairment and dementia in postmenopausal women is not known.

Well-being has been included as a formal outcome in several of the studies of testosterone treatment of HSDD. Overall, no benefit of testosterone on well-being in these studies was demonstrated.[24] Data for effects on mood are limited, but the available data do not support the use of testosterone for the treatment of low mood or depression.[24]

DISCUSSION: PRESCRIBING TESTOSTERONE

Testosterone has been prescribed widely for the treatment of low sexual desire for women for decades.[65–67] Candidates for testosterone therapy are postmenopausal women with HSDD, including women with spontaneous premature ovarian insufficiency and women who have experienced iatrogenic ovarian failure secondary to chemotherapy, radiotherapy, or chemical ovarian suppression.

A diagnosis of HSDD requires a full biopsychosocial assessment, and treatment with testosterone should be considered only when other modifiable factors have been identified and managed.[21] An excellent clinician guide for the assessment of women for HSDD is provided by a process of care developed by the International Society for the Study of Women's Sexual Health.[21] In brief, it is important that each woman is assessed in the context of her personal circumstances, partnership status, sexual experiences, and cultural expectations. It should not be assumed that a woman is experiencing adequate sexual stimulation, both physical and emotional, such that this does need to be explored. Referral to either a psychologist or sexual counselor often is appropriate. Medical history needs to include general medical, psychosocial and uro-gynecological details and the use of all medications, both prescription and nonprescription. A medical examination should include a full genital and pelvic assessment, including assessment of sensitivity in women with loss of sensitivity or sexual pain. Laboratory investigations should be done only as indicated and might include exclusion of factors causing fatigue and hence low sexual interest (iron deficiency and thyroid dysfunction).

Contraindications to testosterone therapy primarily are related to an increased risk of worsening existing acne, hirsutism, and alopecia as well as pregnancy or lactation and hormone-dependent cancer. The large published studies of testosterone for HSDD excluded women with chronic disease; therefore, the safety data generated by these studies cannot be generalized to women with chronic significant health issues. A large, randomized trial of transdermal testosterone versus placebo recruited 3656 postmenopausal women at high risk of cardiometabolic disease.[68] At 4 years, with more than 7000 women-years accrued, the safety monitoring committee had completed 6 unblinded reviews of the data and recommended the study continue. Lack of funding, however, resulted in premature termination of the study. The initial findings have not been shared beyond the safety monitoring committee and the data sit in a repository, unanalyzed. The ethics of this is questionable, in that individual women have had up to 4 years of testosterone therapy without the consequences being evaluated, not only depriving these individual women who committed themselves to this research their results but also depriving women and clinicians across the world research findings that would inform this therapeutic field profoundly.

When testosterone supplementation is indicated, this should be by a transdermal/nonoral testosterone formulation.[2] This is because oral testosterone therapy is associated with lowering of high-density lipoprotein cholesterol and increases in high-density lipoprotein cholesterol.[24] Currently, in most countries, the prescribing of testosterone for women presents a therapeutic challenge because no national regulatory body has approved a testosterone formulation specifically for women. A loose exception to this is Australia, whereby a 1% testosterone transdermal cream has been approved in 1 state and, therefore, legally can be prescribed nationally for women. Specific recommendation of the global consensus was that treatment doses should "approximate physiologic testosterone concentrations for premenopausal women."[2] The global consensus expert panel strongly recommended against the use of testosterone injections, subcutaneous pellets, or any formulation that results in supraphysiologic blood concentrations of testosterone and against compounded preparations.[2] In the United Kingdom, testosterone is available as a testosterone pellet implanted under local anesthetic subcutaneously. These pellets are not compounded individually and a dose of 50 mg mostly is used.[66] The pellets usually remain effective for periods of 4 months to 6 months, although there is considerable intraindividual and interindividual variation in their absorption and degradation.[69] Therefore, repeat implantation should not be undertaken without confirmation that total testosterone corrected for SHBG or free testosterone has fallen into the lower normal female range. Otherwise, the risk of adverse androgenic effects is increased with the insertion of a new implant. Where a regulatory-approved formulation for women is not available, the preferred option is prescription of a fractionated dose of a regulator-approved male formulation.[2] If this is not available, then a compounded testosterone formulation, compliant with purity of active pharmaceutical ingredients and good manufacturing practice to meet industry standards for quality and safety, can be prescribed.[2] Caution is urged, however, because there are no published pharmacokinetic or safety data or efficacy studies to validate or guide the use of compounded formulations.

As discussed previously, there is no blood testosterone concentration that can be used to determine women most likely to benefit from treatment. Clinical trial data have indicated, however, that women with SHBG concentrations above the normal range are less likely to respond to transdermal testosterone.[70] Therefore, before initiating therapy, pretreatment concentrations of SHBG and testosterone should be measured. It is important to recognize that the SHBG concentration also influences the total testosterone concentration. RCTs have shown that women with higher SHBG levels, such as women on oral estrogen, have higher total testosterone for any given transdermal testosterone dose than women with lower baseline SHBG levels, for example, women using transdermal E_2 or no concurrent estrogen therapy.[71–73] Measuring total and free testosterone in women with extremely low SHBG concentrations can be deceptive, because, even with treatment, their blood testosterone remains low because of rapid clearance from the circulation due to the low SHBG.

Studies of transdermal testosterone for HSDD consistently have shown that when a physiologic dose is used, response to treatment can take approximately 4 weeks to 6 weeks.[74] The peak improvement in sexual desire has been seen at approximately 12 weeks, with the nadir in personal distress, and, therefore, reduction in HSDD, at 24 weeks.[74] Therefore, if testosterone is to be prescribed, women need to be advised that they are being given a trial of therapy and that they need to persist with the treatment for several weeks before they can judge whether or not it is beneficial to them. It has been the author's practice, based on clinical experience, to have patients have their testosterone and SHBG levels measured after using the prescribed dose for approximately 3 weeks, to ensure that patients are not applying an excessive dose of testosterone inadvertently, and to review patients after 12 weeks of therapy. If no treatment benefit is seen by 6 months, treatment should by discontinued, because any benefit would have been experienced by this time.[70,72,74,75] Any patients who continue testosterone beyond 6 months should have their testosterone concentration measured regularly, approximately every 6 months, to ensure that they are not applying an excessive dose. The potential masculinizing effects of testosterone therapy include development of acne, hirsutism, deepening of the voice, and androgenic alopecia. These effects are dose related and are uncommon if supraphysiologic hormone levels are avoided. Compared with placebo therapy, women treated with transdermal testosterone in various studies report a higher rate of androgenic adverse events, mainly attributable to increased hair growth.[24] Withdrawal from research studies, however, due to androgenic adverse events, has not been seen to be greater in women treated with testosterone.[72,75] Nonetheless, ongoing users of testosterone must have regular clinical review and be screened for signs of androgen excess.

SUMMARY

Robust clinical trials have shown that, in appropriate doses, testosterone is effective for the treatment of HSDD in postmenopausal women, after exclusion of other modifiable factors. Based on available data, testosterone supplementation should not be used to improve cardiometabolic, musculoskeletal, or cognitive health or well-being and low mood in postmenopausal women.

Regulatory approval of testosterone formulations for women urgently is needed so that women who meet the criteria for treatment have access to a reliable, regulated treatment. This protects women from inappropriate dosing with substitute compounded and male formulations. There also is a pressing need for more research into testosterone therapy for women, including fracture prevention, maintenance of cognitive function and of CV and mental health, and long-term safety of use.

CLINICS CARE POINTS

- A diagnosis of HSDD requires a comprehensive clinical biopsychosocial assessment.
- Dosing is not based on testosterone blood levels; there is no blood testosterone concentration target to achieve with treatment; and supraphysiologic testosterone concentrations should be avoided.
- It is important to ensure women treated with testosterone understand that they are having a therapeutic trial, that treatment benefits may not be experienced for several weeks when a physiologic dose is prescribed, and that not all treated patients benefit.
- Although compounded subcutaneous testosterone implants with/without concurrent aromatase inhibitor implants are being promoted to treat/prevent breast cancer, the safety and efficacy of this approach have not been evaluated in an appropriate placebo-controlled RCT.
- Because currently available testosterone formulations require patients to measure out each dose to be applied, it is essential that treated patients are evaluated regularly for clinical signs and biochemical concentrations consistent with androgen excess.
- Although available data indicate physiologic testosterone supplementation to be safe, the long-term safety of testosterone therapy for women has yet to be established.

DISCLOSURES

Dr S.R. Davis reports having received honoraria from BioFemme, Besins Healthcare, and Pfizer Australia. She has also been a consultant to Mayne Pharmaceuticals, Lawley Pharmaceuticals, Roche Pharmaceuticals, Que Oncology, Abbott Pharmaceuticals, and Astellas Pharmaceuticals.

REFERENCES

1. Simpson ER, Davis SR. Minireview: aromatase and the regulation of estrogen biosynthesis–some new perspectives. Endocrinology 2001;142:4589–94.
2. Davis SR, Baber R, Panay N, et al. Global consensus position statement on the use of testosterone therapy for women. Climacteric 2019;22:429–34.
3. Davis SR, Wahlin-Jacobsen S. Testosterone in women–the clinical significance. Lancet Diabetes Endocrinol 2015;3:980–92.

4. Skiba MA, Bell RJ, Islam RM, et al. Androgens during the reproductive years, what's normal for women? J Clin Endocrinol Metab 2019;104(11):5382–92.
5. Dunn JF, Nisula BC, Rodboard D. Transport of steroid hormones. Binding of 21 endogenous steroids to both testosterone-binding globulin and cortico-steroid-binding globulin in human plasma. J Clin Endocrinol Metab 1981;53:58–68.
6. Handelsman DJ. Free testosterone: pumping up the tires or ending the free ride? Endocr Rev 2017;38:297–301.
7. Goldman AL, Bhasin S, Wu FCW, et al. A reappraisal of testosterone's binding in circulation: physiological and clinical implications. Endocr Rev 2017;38:302–24.
8. Rosner W, Vesper H. Toward excellence in testosterone testing: a consensus statement. J Clin Endocrinol Metab 2010;95:4542–8.
9. Nestler JE, Strauss JF 3rd. Insulin as an effector of human ovarian and adrenal steroid metabolism. Endocrinol Metab Clin North Am 1991;20:807–23.
10. Goodman-Gruen D, Barrett-Connor E. Sex hormone-binding globulin and glucose tolerance in postmenopausal women. The rancho Bernardo study. Diabetes Care 1997;20:645–9.
11. Randolph JF Jr, Sowers M, Gold EB, et al. Reproductive hormones in the early menopausal transition: relationship to ethnicity, body size, and menopausal status. J Clin Endocrinol Metab 2003;88:1516–22.
12. Ding EL, Song Y, Manson JE, et al. Sex hormone-binding globulin and risk of type 2 diabetes in women and men. N Engl J Med 2009;361:1152–63.
13. Davis SR, Robinson PJ, Moufarege A, et al. The contribution of SHBG to the variation in HOMA-IR is not dependent on endogenous oestrogen or androgen levels in postmenopausal women. Clin Endocrinol (Oxf) 2012;77:541–7.
14. Janssen I, Powell LH, Kazlauskaite R, et al. Testosterone and visceral fat in midlife women: the Study of Women's Health Across the Nation (SWAN) fat patterning study. Obesity (Silver Spring) 2010;18:604–10.
15. Golden SH, Dobs AS, Vaidya D, et al. Endogenous sex hormones and glucose tolerance status in postmenopausal women. J Clin Endocrinol Metab 2007;92:1289–95.
16. Labrie F. Intracrinology. Mol Cell Endocrinol 1991;78:C113–8.
17. Wahlin-Jacobsen S, Pedersen AT, Kristensen E, et al. Is there a correlation between androgens and sexual desire in women? J Sex Med 2014;12(2):358–73.
18. Davison SL, Bell R, Donath S, et al. Androgen levels in adult females: changes with age, menopause, and oophorectomy. J Clin Endocrinol Metab 2005;90:3847–53.
19. Zheng J, Islam MR, Skiba MA, et al. Associations between androgens and sexual function in premenopausal women: a cross-sectional study. Lancet Diabetes Endocrinol 2020;8(8):693–702.
20. Randolph JF Jr, Zheng H, Avis NE, et al. Masturbation frequency and sexual function domains are associated with serum reproductive hormone levels across the menopausal transition. J Clin Endocrinol Metab 2015;100:258–66.
21. Clayton AH, Goldstein I, Kim NN, et al. The international society for the study of women's sexual health process of care for management of hypoactive sexual desire disorder in women. Mayo Clin Proc 2018;93:467–87.
22. Zheng J, Skiba MA, Bell RJ, et al. The prevalence of sexual dysfunction and sexually-related distress in young women: a cross-sectional survey. Fertil Steril 2020;113(2):426–34.
23. Worsley R, Bell RJ, Gartoulla P, et al. Prevalence and predictors of low sexual desire, sexually related personal distress, and hypoactive sexual desire dysfunction in a community-based sample of midlife women. J Sex Med 2017;14:675–86.

24. Islam RM, Bell RJ, Green S, et al. Safety and efficacy of testosterone for women: a systematic review and meta-analysis of randomised controlled trial data. Lancet Diabetes Endocrinol 2019;7:754–66.

25. Archer JS, Love-Geffen TE, Herbst-Damm KL, et al. Effect of estradiol versus estradiol and testosterone on brain-activation patterns in postmenopausal women. Menopause 2006;13:528–37.

26. Baldassarre M, Perrone AM, Giannone FA, et al. Androgen receptor expression in the human vagina under different physiological and treatment conditions. Int J Impot Res 2013;25:7–11.

27. Heard-Davison A, Heiman JR, Kuffel S. Genital and subjective measurement of the time course effects of an acute dose of testosterone vs. placebo in postmenopausal women. J Sex Med 2007;4:209–17.

28. Salinger SL. Proliferative effect of testosterone propionate on human vaginal epithelium. Acta Endocrinol (Copenh) 1950;4:265–84.

29. Bell RJ, Rizvi F, Islam RM, et al. A systematic review of intravaginal testosterone for the treatment of vulvovaginal atrophy. Menopause 2018;25:704–9.

30. Witherby S, Johnson J, Demers L, et al. Topical testosterone for breast cancer patients with vaginal atrophy related to aromatase inhibitors: a phase I/II study. Oncologist 2011;16:424–31.

31. Dahir M, Travers-Gustafson D. Breast cancer, aromatase inhibitor therapy, and sexual functioning: a pilot study of the effects of vaginal testosterone therapy. Sex Med 2014;2:8–15.

32. Raghunandan C, Agrawal S, Dubey P, et al. A comparative study of the effects of local estrogen with or without local testosterone on vulvovaginal and sexual dysfunction in postmenopausal women. J Sex Med 2010;7:1284–90.

33. Fernandes T, Costa-Paiva LH, Pinto-Neto AM. Efficacy of vaginally applied estrogen, testosterone, or polyacrylic acid on sexual function in postmenopausal women: a randomized controlled trial. J Sex Med 2014;11:1262–70.

34. Melisko ME, Goldman ME, Hwang J, et al. Vaginal testosterone cream vs estradiol vaginal ring for vaginal dryness or decreased libido in women receiving aromatase inhibitors for early-stage breast cancer: a randomized clinical trial. JAMA Oncol 2017;3:313–9.

35. Davis SR: Supplementary data-Intra-vaginal testosterone improves sexual satisfaction and vaginal symptoms associated with aromatase inhibitors. 2018.pdf. figshare. Dataset. 2018; https://doi.org/10.26180/5b6517ab522f4.

36. Mitchell KR, Mercer CH, Ploubidis GB, et al. Sexual function in Britain: findings from the third national survey of sexual attitudes and lifestyles (Natsal-3). Lancet 2013;382:1817–29.

37. Barlow DH. Causes of sexual dysfunction: the role of anxiety and cognitive interference. J Consult Clin Psychol 1986;54:140–8.

38. Stephenson KR, Meston CM. Why is impaired sexual function distressing to women? The primacy of pleasure in female sexual dysfunction. J Sex Med 2015;12:728–37.

39. Hayes RD, Dennerstein L, Bennett CM, et al. Relationship between hypoactive sexual desire disorder and aging. Fertil Steril 2007;87:107–12.

40. Shifren JL, Monz BU, Russo PA, et al. Sexual problems and distress in United States women: prevalence and correlates. Obstet Gynecol 2008;112:970–8.

41. West SL, D'Aloisio AA, Agans RP, et al. Prevalence of low sexual desire and hypoactive sexual desire disorder in a nationally representative sample of US women. Arch Intern Med 2008;168:1441–9.

42. Zeleke B, Bell RJ, Billah B, et al. Hypoactive sexual desire dysfunction in community-dwelling older women. Menopause 2016;24(4):391–9.
43. Spoletini I, Vitale C, Pelliccia F, et al. Androgens and cardiovascular disease in postmenopausal women: a systematic review. Climacteric 2014;17:625–34.
44. Jones RD, Hugh Jones T, Channer KS. The influence of testosterone upon vascular reactivity. Eur J Endocrinol 2004;151:29–37.
45. Worboys S, Kotsopoulos D, Teede H, et al. Parental testosterone improves endothelium-dependent and independent vasodilation in postmenopausal women already receiving estrogen. J Clin Endocrinol Metab 2001;86:158–61.
46. Montalcini T, Gorgone G, Gazzaruso C, et al. Endogenous testosterone and endothelial function in postmenopausal women. Coron Artery Dis 2007;18:9–13.
47. Navarro-Dorado J, Orensanz LM, Recio P, et al. Mechanisms involved in testosterone-induced vasodilatation in pig prostatic small arteries. Life Sci 2008;83:569–73.
48. Davison S, Thipphawong J, Blanchard J, et al. Pharmacokinetics and acute safety of inhaled testosterone in postmenopausal women. J Clin Pharmacol 2005;45:177–84.
49. Bidoggia H, Maciel JP, Capalozza N, et al. Sex differences on the electrocardiographic pattern of cardiac repolarization: possible role of testosterone. Am Heart J 2000;140:678–83.
50. Dunlay SM, Roger VL. Gender differences in the pathophysiology, clinical presentation, and outcomes of ischemic heart failure. Curr Heart Fail Rep 2012;9: 267–76.
51. Schaffrath G, Kische H, Gross S, et al. Association of sex hormones with incident 10-year cardiovascular disease and mortality in women. Maturitas 2015;82: 424–30.
52. Sievers C, Klotsche J, Pieper L, et al. Low testosterone levels predict all-cause mortality and cardiovascular events in women: a prospective cohort study in German primary care patients. Eur J Endocrinol 2010;163:699–708.
53. Laughlin GA, Goodell V, Barrett-Connor E. Extremes of endogenous testosterone are associated with increased risk of incident coronary events in older women. J Clin Endocrinol Metab 2010;95:740–7.
54. Benn M, Voss SS, Holmegard HN, et al. Extreme concentrations of endogenous sex hormones, ischemic heart disease, and death in women. Arterioscler Thromb Vasc Biol 2015;35:471–7.
55. Lellamo F, Volterrani M, Caminiti G, et al. Testosterone therapy in women with chronic heart failure: a pilot double-blind, randomized, placebo-controlled study. J Am Coll Cardiol 2010;56:1310–6.
56. Saki F, Kasaee SR, Sadeghian F, et al. The effect of testosterone itself and in combination with letrozole on bone mineral density in male rats. J Bone Miner Metab 2019;37:668–75.
57. Rariy CM, Ratcliffe SJ, Weinstein R, et al. Higher serum free testosterone concentration in older women is associated with greater bone mineral density, lean body mass, and total fat mass: the cardiovascular health study. J Clin Endocrinol Metab 2011;96:989–96.
58. Lee JS, LaCroix AZ, Wu L, et al. Associations of serum sex hormone-binding globulin and sex hormone concentrations with hip fracture risk in postmenopausal women. J Clin Endocrinol Metab 2008;93:1796–803.
59. Yuki A, Ando F, Otsuka R, et al. Low free testosterone is associated with loss of appendicular muscle mass in Japanese community-dwelling women. Geriatr Gerontol Int 2015;15:326–33.

60. Pike CJ, Carroll JC, Rosario ER, et al. Protective actions of sex steroid hormones in Alzheimer's disease. Front Neuroendocrinol 2009;30:239–58.
61. Drake EB, Henderson VW, Stanczyk FZ, et al. Associations between circulating sex steroid hormones and cognition in normal elderly women. Neurology 2000; 54:599–603.
62. Wolf OT, Kirschbaum C. Endogenous estradiol and testosterone levels are associated with cognitive performance in older women and men. Horm Behav 2002; 41:259.
63. Shah SM, Bell RJ, Savage G, et al. Testosterone aromatization and cognition in women: a randomized placebo controlled trial. Menopause 2006;13:600–8.
64. Davis SR, Jane F, Robinson PJ, et al. Transdermal testosterone improves verbal learning and memory in postmenopausal women not on oestrogen therapy. Clin Endocrinol (Oxf) 2014;81:621–8.
65. Burger HG, Hailes J, Menelaus M. The management of persistent symptoms with estradiol-testosterone implants: clinical, lipid and hormonal results. Maturitas 1984;6:351.
66. Davis SR, McCloud PI, Strauss BJG, et al. Testosterone enhances estradiol's effects on postmenopausal bone density and sexuality. Maturitas 1995;21:227–36.
67. Greenblatt RB. Testosterone proprionate pellet implanation in gyneic disorders. JAMA 1943;121:17–24.
68. White WB, Grady D, Giudice LC, et al. A cardiovascular safety study of LibiGel (testosterone gel) in postmenopausal women with elevated cardiovascular risk and hypoactive sexual desire disorder. Am Heart J 2012;163:27–32.
69. Buckler HM, Kalsi PK, Cantrill JA, et al. An audit of oestradiol levels and implant frequency in women undergoing subcutaneous implant therapy. Clin Endocrinol (Oxf) 1995;42:445–50.
70. Shifren J, Davis SR, Moreau M, et al. Testosterone patch for the treatment of hypoactive sexual desire disorder in naturally menopausal women: results from the INTIMATE NM1 study. Menopause 2006;13:770–9.
71. Davis SR, van der Mooren MJ, van Lunsen RHW, et al. The efficacy and safety of a testosterone patch for the treatment of hypoactive sexual desire disorder in surgically menopausal women: a randomized, placebo-controlled trial. Menopause 2006;13:387–96.
72. Davis SR, Moreau M, Kroll R, et al. Testosterone for low libido in menopausal women not taking estrogen therapy. N Engl J Med 2008;359:2005–17.
73. Braunstein G, Shifren J, Simon J, Lucas J, Rodenberg C, Watts NB: Testosterone patches for the treatment of low sexual desire in surgically menopausal women. Proceedings of the 14th Annual Meeting of the North American Menopause Society. Miami (FL), September 18-20, 2003.
74. Advisory Committee Briefing Document Intrinsa® (testosterone transdermal system) 2 December 2004. NDA No. 21-769 Procter & Gamble Pharmaceuticals, Inc. Advisory Committee for Reproductive Health Drugs. 2009. 2019. Available at: https://wayback.archive-it.org/7993/20170405114619/https://www.fda.gov/ohrms/dockets/ac/04/briefing/2004-4082B1_01_A-P&G-Intrinsa.pdf. Accessed April 20, 2019.
75. Panay N, Al-Azzawi F, Bouchard C, et al. Testosterone treatment of HSDD in naturally menopausal women: the ADORE study. Climacteric 2010;13:121–31.

Sexual Dysfunctions in Women: Are Androgens at Fault?

Rosemary Basson, MD, FRCP(UK)*

KEYWORDS

- Women's sexual dysfunctions • Androgens • Intracrine • Cognitive therapy

KEY POINTS

- Current evidence does not support androgen deficiency as a cause of women's sexual dysfunctions: it is not recommended to measure serum androgens or metabolites when investigating these disorders.
- Supplemental testosterone has not been trialed in women with sexual disorders as currently defined.
- Many aspects of androgen activity remain to be investigated for any modulation of women's sexual function, for example, neurosteroids, variations in androgen receptor sensitivity, and androgen metabolites acting independent of the androgen receptor.
- Before and after menopause, in health and in chronic disease, psychosocial factors are robustly associated with women's sexual dysfunctions.
- Management focuses on clarifying where a woman's personal, interpersonal, and contextual factors interfere with her sex response cycle to understand the cause of her sexual dysfunction and indicate management options.

INTRODUCTION
What Constitutes Sexual Dysfunction?

That women's sexual experiences are often problematic is rarely disputed, but when those experiences should be termed dysfunctional remains uncertain. There are 3 female sexual disorders listed in the 2013 American Psychiatric Association's (APA) *Diagnostic and Statistical Manual of Mental Disorders* (Fifth Edition; *DSM-5*)[1] that focus on painful sex, orgasm difficulty, and insufficient sexual arousal and interest, that is, sexual interest and arousal disorder (SIAD).

The role of androgens has been investigated in low sexual desire. SIAD replaced the former *DSM-IV-Text Revised* (APA 2000)[2] diagnosis of female hypoactive sexual desire disorder (HSDD), the diagnostic criteria of which focused on frequency of sexual fantasy and of desire for sexual activity. Long-standing criticism of a focus on

Conflict of interest: The author has no conflict of interest.
Department of Psychiatry, University of British Columbia, Vancouver, British Columbia, Canada
* BC Centre for Sexual Medicine, 818 West 10th Avenue, Vancouver, British Columbia V5Z 1M9, Canada.
E-mail address: bassonreees@telus.net

Endocrinol Metab Clin N Am 50 (2021) 125–138
https://doi.org/10.1016/j.ecl.2020.12.001   endo.theclinics.com
0889-8529/21/© 2020 Elsevier Inc. All rights reserved.

fantasies as a measure of women's sexual desire and of the underlying assumption that healthy desire is necessarily experienced ahead of sexual engagement (for review, see Brotto[3]) led to an evidenced-based definition of SIAD with 6 possible components: no or rare sexual interest, sexual thoughts, sexual activity, sexual pleasure when sexually active, no experience of desire once aroused (responsive desire), and loss of genital sexual sensitivity. If at least 3 of the 6 are troublesome to the woman and last more than 6 months, a diagnosis of SIAD is likely.

Sexual desire at the outset of sexual activity may not be the predominant type of desire experienced by women.[4] Women frequently identify a "triggered" or "responsive" sexual desire along with arousal in response to sexual stimuli.[5–8] In addition to reflecting the importance of responsive desire, SIAD criteria also include lack of pleasure, lack of subjective arousal, that is, "excitement,"[9] and reduced physical sexual sensations.

Criticism of the SIAD diagnostic criteria includes the lack of continuity with previous versions of the *DSM*[10–13] and that its stricter criteria "unfairly raised the bar" for a diagnosis of sexual desire disorder.[12] A systematic comparison has since clarified that 73.5% of women who meet criteria for HSDD also maintain a clinical diagnosis of SIAD.[14] The 26.5% of women meeting criteria for HSDD only reported significantly higher sexual satisfaction, receptivity to sexual invitations, more frequent sexual desire, more positive sexual thoughts, more responsivity to erotica, easier sexual arousal, more desire following sexual arousal, as well as easier orgasms. Only 7% of women with HSDD but not SIAD reported lack of pleasure or lack of physical sexual sensations to at least a moderate degree. These results from systematic comparison of SIAD and HSDD highlights the difficulties in interpreting the benefit for HSDD afforded by some of the testosterone trials to a likely benefit for SIAD.

A Sex Hormonal Basis for Women's Sexual Dysfunction

A hormonal basis for women's sexual dysfunction has long been suspected. Menopause and stages of the menstrual cycle frequently impact sexual function and desire.[15,16] However, aside from estrogen deficit-related genital changes, which may reduce intensity of sexual sensations, vaginal lubrication, and coital comfort, the larger role of sex hormones in women's sexual disorders remains elusive.

That androgen deficit underlies women's sexual dysfunction has been suspected for more than half a century and remains a focus of research.[17–21] Although an "androgen deficiency disease" has never been identified, nor have trials of testosterone supplementation in women with sexual dysfunction included any measure of androgen deficit, there remains ongoing off-label prescription of supplemental testosterone for women's sexual dysfunction.

Recent meta-analyses of randomized controlled trials (RCTs) of transdermal systemic testosterone supplementation conclude that such prescription is "effective for postmenopausal women with low sexual desire causing distress."[22] Because negative trials of similar testosterone supplementation are published only in abstract form,[23] they are excluded in meta-analyses. The RCTs predated current definitions of sexual disorders, thereby questioning the presence of baseline dysfunction of recruited women.

There are many reasons to seriously question "are androgens at fault" and to question androgen supplementation, including those in **Box 1**.

HISTORY

Unintended sexual effects increasing sexual desire or "libido" from highly supraphysiologic doses of testosterone given for advanced breast cancer were noted some

8 decades ago.[26] Subsequent noncontrolled trials of supplemental supraphysiologic testosterone followed. Despite findings that estrogen plus testosterone was more effective in increasing sexual desire than testosterone-alone testosterone, supplementation for "low libido" was pursued. More recent research aimed to supplement testosterone in postmenopausal women to reach high normal premenopausal levels, although some supraphysiologic levels were identified.[27]

BACKGROUND
Major Confounds to the Question "Are Androgens at Fault"

The following entities repeatedly hamper clarity on the role of androgens in women's sexuality.

Intracrine sources of androgen
Before menopause, some 50%, and after menopause, near 100%, of testosterone in tissues are derived from adrenal precursors, including dehydroepiandrosterone (DHEA). The amount produced in this intracrine manner cannot be measured directly. Androgen metabolites reflect intracrine production, and to date, androsterone glucuronide has been considered the most useful metabolite to measure.[28] Only more recent studies have included this measurement.

Inaccurate serum testosterone assays
Free testosterone levels in women can be measured by radioimmunoassay; however, the accuracy at testosterone levels less than 300 ng/dL is limited.[29] Nonextraction radioimmunoassay for measurement of total testosterone was widely used, but is unreliable in women.[29] The more accurate gas/liquid chromatography–mass spectrometry assays have only recently become available.[28]

Lack of validated questionnaires assessing women's sexual disorders using Diagnostic and Statistical Manual of Mental Disorders (fifth edition) criteria
The Female Sexual Function Index (FSFI) is frequently used in the research literature to assess women's sexual desire and dysfunction, despite its intended use to monitor treatment. Because the FSFI is based on *DSM-IV* HSDD, the criticism of HSDD applies to the FSFI.

Aspects of androgen activity yet unexplored in relationship to sexual function
The roles of brain-derived androgens, that is, neurosteroids, androgen receptor sensitivity, and possible active androgen metabolites, remain largely unexplored in the area of sexual function.

EXAMINING EVIDENCE IN SUPPORT OF A ROLE OF ANDROGENS IN WOMEN'S SEXUAL DYSFUNCTION

Despite the long-standing "belief" that androgen deficit underlies some of women's sexual dysfunction, to date, there is no confirmation of this. Confirmation was predicted when researchers were able to measure androgen metabolites to reflect total androgen activity, including that from intracrine production. However, women (and their partners if in long-term relationships) assessed by both interview and validated questionnaires detected no difference in androgens as measured by serum testosterone or testosterone metabolites between 150 women with HSDD and 150 controls.[17] **Table 1** provides a critique of evidence supporting a role for androgens in women's sexual dysfunction.

EXAMINING EVIDENCE AGAINST ANDROGEN'S ROLE IN WOMEN'S SEXUAL DYSFUNCTION

Although a strong argument can be made for a lack of androgen's role in the clinical presentation of low desire dating from menopause when androgen production changes minimally, the research is limited. **Table 2** provides a critique of the evidence refuting a role for androgens in women's sexual dysfunction.

SEXUAL DESIRE AND DEHYDROEPIANDROSTERONE

Many studies have shown an association between low sexual desire and low serum DHEA.[17,18,21,43] DHEA has multiple actions in the brain, but the clinical significance remains unclear save from its effect to improve mood. In other words, it is possible that this "preandrogen" might underlie some sexual dysfunction, but not via its androgenic potential. However, it is also possible that the low DHEA is simply a marker of hypothalamic pituitary adrenal (HPA) dysregulation in keeping with recent work finding low DHEA levels and other parameters of such dysregulation to be present in women with low sexual desire in comparison to control women.[17,18] An additional explanation is that low DHEA, possibly from HPA axis dysregulation, affects desire via its potential to influence mood.

IS ANY SEX HORMONE AT FAULT?

The sudden drop in estrogen at menopause and the identified loss of sexual desire in many women at this time suggest a role for estrogen to foster sexual desire. For reasons of safety, menopausal estrogen therapy is not administered to periovulatory levels such that it is possible that simultaneous supplemental testosterone is of benefit primarily from its conversion to estrogen by aromatization. Meta-analyses of sex hormone supplementation to treat postmenopausal sexual dysfunction before the more recent studies of transdermal testosterone concluded that some estrogen-alone therapies were associated with an improvement in women's sexual function, but that androgen therapies were only effective when administered in combination with an estrogen.[47] A 2016 meta-analysis[27] found that 4 of the 5 estrogen-only older studies, which achieved levels of estradiol similar to those around ovulation, increased sexual desire in postmenopausal women. Some of the studies involving currently approved menopausal estrogen therapy plus testosterone therapy led to modest increase in sexual desire, but invoked supraphysiologic testosterone.[42,48,49] The investigators suggest the improved effectiveness of an estrogen in combination with supraphysiologic testosterone "may reflect testosterone's aromatization to estradiol and/or the dynamic relationship between estradiol, testosterone and SHBG."[27]

Table 1
Critique of evidence supporting a role for androgens in women's sexual dysfunction

Condition/Argument	Supporting Evidence	Critique
Premature surgical menopause	Increased prevalence of *distress* regarding low sexual desire after a recent bilateral salpingo-oophorectomy (BSO)[31]	After BSO, women reported similar levels of low sexual desire to age-matched subjects with intact ovaries. With nonelective surgery, the thematic context of BSO may impair sexual desire to a distressing degree[31]
		Sexual dysfunction is not reported after elective surgery for benign disease[30]
		Sexual ideation is similar in women with or without BSO[32]
Research in women with nonclassic congenital adrenal hyperplasia (NCCAH) is limited	A recent study of 24 women with NCCAH reported higher sexual desire than controls[33]	Women with NCCAH had a *lower* total FSFI score, with lower sexual arousal, lubrication, sexual satisfaction[33]
Midcycle peaks of sexual desire and testosterone	Past research supports increased sexual activity at midcycle[34]	More recent research confirmed a midcycle peak in desire, but no effects of changes in salivary testosterone after controlling for estradiol and progesterone levels[34]
Oral combined contraceptives	An unknown percentage of women using oral combined contraceptives reports reduced sexual desire often attributed to the estrogen component, increasing sex hormone-binding globulin (SHBG), thereby reducing free testosterone	When oral DHEA is added to contraceptive regimens, results are conflicting.[35,36] The relevance of any reduction of free testosterone by estrogen effect on SHBG has been questioned.[21] The precise percentage of women experiencing loss of desire from the combined pill is unclear, but this effect would appear to be limited

(continued on next page)

Table 1
(continued)

Condition/Argument	Supporting Evidence	Critique
Testosterone supplementation to postmenopausal women with sexual complaints	RCTs of transdermal testosterone supplementation to (mostly surgically) postmenopausal women[22,23,37,38] give conflicting results, but benefit was documented when the transdermal patch formulation (but not the gel formulation achieving similar serum testosterone levels) was used	The RCTs did not identify baseline deficit[39,50,51] Questionable baseline dysfunction: Is having 2–3 sexually satisfying experiences per month[39] dysfunctional? Some testosterone levels were supraphysiologic[27] Treatment benefit was assessed using a questionnaire based on prior criteria of disorder[39]
Testosterone supplementation to postmenopausal women with low serum testosterone but without sexual complaints	For women receiving estrogen therapy who had serum testosterone <31 ng/dL supplementing with either 3, 6.25, 12.5, or 25 mg intramuscular testosterone weekly increased sexual thoughts, fantasies, and sexual activity (but not receptivity, initiation, or pleasure), in only the 25-mg group[40]	All doses lead to moderate or excessively supraphysiologic levels of testosterone
Supplemental testosterone in the absence of supplemental estrogen to menopausal women	Testosterone given to postmenopausal women with low desire in the absence of supplemental estrogen has shown some benefit[41,42]	Markedly supraphysiologic levels of testosterone in the older study and more modest supraphysiologic levels (>60 ng/dL) in the later study[42] implies that only supraphysiologic levels of testosterone can increase sexual desire in estrogen-deficient postmenopausal women

Data from Refs. [21–23,27,30–42,50,51]

Table 2
Critique of evidence refuting a role for androgens in women's sexual dysfunction

Condition/Argument	Supporting Evidence	Critique
Low desire after natural menopause is common,[24] but androgen production changes minimally	Intracrine testosterone continues to slowly decline from late 30s to early 60s. Ovarian production of testosterone does not change significantly at menopause	Research comparing testosterone levels in women with and without a menopausal marked loss in desire using mass spectrometry assays has not been done
Paucity of evidence associating sexual dysfunction with androgen deficiency	Neither large epidemiologic studies[43] nor recent studies using markers of intracrine androgen & mass spectrometry methods have linked sexual desire to serum androgen levels[17,20,21]	Research typically excludes women with treated or untreated depression (most women complaining of low desire). Could androgen deficiency act in synergy with low mood to reduce desire?
Women with complete androgen deficiency syndrome (CAIS) can have healthy sexual desire and response	Despite psychosocial issues, including infertility, delay in disclosure, reduced sexual confidence, and increased risk of depression, women with CAIS can be sexually functional[44]	Androgen relevance is not entirely precluded by androgen receptor resistance. For instance, an androgen metabolite could be acting via non-receptor-mediated mechanisms
Polycystic ovarian syndrome (PCOS) is not associated with high desire	Women with naturally high testosterone levels as in PCOS do not report heightened sexual desire compared with controls[45,46]	Studies focused on women with PCOS but without untoward effects of high testosterone on weight, hirsutism, and alopecia are needed

Data from Refs.[17,20,21,24,43–46]

NEEDED RESEARCH

There are several areas of research that remain largely unexplored, but are needed in order to answer the question, "Are androgens at fault?"

1. What is the role of androgens in sexual dysfunction per se, that is, not only dysfunction that causes the woman to be distressed (although this subgroup is the clinically important one)?
2. What is the role of androgens over and beyond that reflected by serum levels or independent of their action through the androgen receptor (**Table 3**)?
3. Loss of genital sexual sensitivity. An unknown number of women reporting low desire at menopause state that their desire was formerly felt physically, and it is that physical/genital aspect they have lost. Orgasms typically are muted or absent. This potential menopausal change of lost genital sexual sensitivity is now included in *DSM-5*'s definition of SIAD. There is early evidence that testosterone may be important for genital sexual sensitivity, and that sensitivity may in some women be an important confirmation and reinforcement of sexual desire.[55] Vaginal DHEA, thought to act locally by its conversion to testosterone and estrogen, has recently been approved for vaginal dryness and pain from postmenopausal genital changes.[55] Studies recruited women with vaginal dryness and pain from the estrogen deficit as opposed to women with lost genital arousal or difficulty with orgasm, but did report improvement in participants' orgasms and increased desire. Further research is needed in the use of vaginal DHEA to restore lost genital arousal.

HOW IS SEXUAL INTEREST/AROUSAL DISORDER ASSESSED AND TREATED?

In contrast to the uncertainty of hormonal influence on desire, sexual arousal, and sexual pleasure, there is robust evidence linking to mood and the interpersonal sexual

Table 3
Androgen function over and beyond that reflected by serum levels

Factors Modulating Androgen Activity	(Limited) Research to Date
Ketosteroids may be relevant active androgens: androgenic steroid 11-ketotestosterone & 11-ketodihydrotestosterone can activate androgen receptor signaling[50]	Cross-sectional analysis of 588 premenopausal women found no significant associations between serum testosterone, 11-ketoandrostenedione, or 11-ketotestosterone and sexual function[21]
Other active androgen metabolites acting in ways other than on the androgen receptor	Possibly increased efficacy of testosterone therapy over estrogen therapy given to women with complete androgen insensitivity syndrome[51]
Androgen receptor sensitivity	Higher numbers of Cytosine, Adenine, Guanine (CAG) repeats in women reporting more severe pain with intercourse[52] Alternative splice variants in the AR gene associated with enhanced transcription of genes involved in androgen metabolism in women with PCOS[53] but not yet studied in relation to sexual dysfunction
Neurosteroids, including androgen (and/or estrogen) entering the brain from the serum or being produced in the brain,[54] may be more relevant than serum levels	No studies relating to sexual dysfunction

Data from Refs.[21,50–54]

relationship.[56–58] Even in the context of serious chronic illness, depression is an independent risk factor.[59] Thus, assessing and addressing mental health concerns and relationship disharmony is necessary before focusing on details of the woman's sexual response.

Clarifying current understanding of sex response cycles and places of its interruption in the patient forms the basis of assessment.

HUMAN SEX RESPONSE CYCLE

At the outset of a sexual experience, a woman may already sense a degree of sexual arousal and desire for more. However, often women (and men) are motivated by factors other than sexual desire. Research identifies many reasons, including those related to emotional intimacy with their partners.[9,60] By directing one's attention to sexual stimulation, subjective sexual arousal (sexual excitement), with or without conscious awareness of genital arousal, triggers sexual desire. Desire and arousal coexist, compound each other, and are indistinguishable for many women (**Fig. 1**). Sexual satisfaction (with one, many, or no orgasms) can follow by staying focused, providing that pleasure continues, that the duration of the stimulation is sufficiently long, and that there is no negative outcome expected (eg, pain or partner dysfunction).

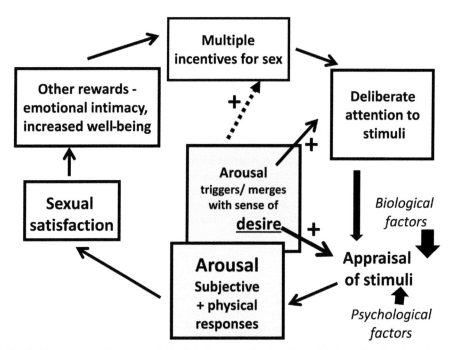

Fig. 1. Human sexual response is depicted as a motivation/incentive-based cycle of overlapping phases of variable order. Desire can be triggered alongside the sexual arousal resulting from attending to sexual stimuli. Sometimes, just anticipating sex is sufficient to trigger arousal and desire such that desire is felt at the outset of sexual activity. Psychological and biological factors influence the brain's appraisal of the sexual stimuli. Arousal will then influence the choice of stimuli and the mind's processing of the same. Sexual and nonsexual outcomes influence present and future sexual motivation. (*Adapted from* Basson R. The female sexual response: the role of drugs in the management of sexual dysfunction. Obstet Gynecol 2001;98:350-352; with permission.)

The response is circular, with phases overlapping and in variable order (eg, desire may follow arousal, and higher arousal may follow the first orgasm).[61–63] Desire, once triggered, increases the motivation to respond to sexual stimuli and to agree to or ask for more intensely erotic forms of stimulation. This motivation/incentives module reflecting the importance of the mind's appraisal of sexual stimuli is supported by empirical research.[64,65] Functional brain imaging during sexual arousal supports an incentive-based model of sexual response showing that multiple areas of the brain are involved. Complex brain circuitry is identified, including cortical, limbic, and paralimbic areas known to be involved in cognition, motivation, and emotions linked to changes within the autonomic nervous system.[61] Specific inhibitory regions deactivate during sexual responses.

Often women relate to difficulties at many sites in the cycle. Personal factors, including low sexual confidence, feeling insufficient connection to her partner, fatigue, finding little reward from her sexual experiences, all frequently lessen a woman's motivation. Lack of needed stimuli and appropriate environment often with limited guidance to her partner for the stimulation needed in that moment may all contribute. Difficulties staying focused often expressed as "having too busy a mind" are common.

In addition to explaining the cycle and its interruptions, clinicians may wish to refer patients to psychologists, physicians with special interest in sexual medicine, or to sex therapists for further treatment. Modalities include cognitive therapy, both traditional and mindfulness-based, and sex therapy, which can assist sexual communication as well as providing needed information.[66–68] Mindfulness-based cognitive therapy is proving to be particularly beneficial for women's difficulties staying present and not worrying about the outcome or self-monitoring their sexual response. If the outcome is expected to be negative, for example, because of pain or partner dysfunction, then these must be addressed initially.

SUMMARY

Evidence that androgen deficiency underlies women's sexual dysfunction is lacking. Limited data support that testosterone therapy may increase desire, but any role in treating currently accepted definitions of sexual disorders is yet untested. However, many aspects of androgen activity remain to be investigated as to their possible modulation of women's sexual function that is, however, robustly linked to psychosocial determinants.

CLINICS CARE POINTS

- Available evidence does not support androgen deficiency as a cause of women's sexual dysfunction. There is no clinical value in measuring serum androgens or metabolites when investigating women's sexual complaints.
- Supplementing testosterone to women with sexual dysfunction as currently defined has not been studied. Past trials recruited women reporting at least some rewarding sexual experiences each month.
- Although there is early limited evidence that vaginal DHEA may improve postmenopausal loss of genital sexual sensitivity, presumably from local conversion to testosterone and estrogen, there is no definitive study: its use for this condition is investigational.
- It remains possible the estrogen deficit is "at fault" for some loss of desire after menopause. This will remain unknown unless a suitable selective estrogen receptor modulator is discovered that mirrors estrogen's activity in the brain before

menopause but does not have estrogen's untoward effects on the endometrium, breast, and coagulation.

- Before and after menopause, in health and in chronic disease, psychosocial factors are robustly associated with women's sexual dysfunctions.
- Once any mental health or relationship issues are addressed, modalities of treatment for sexual dysfunction include explanation of the human sexual response cycle and clarification of areas that are problematic for the particular woman, cognitive therapies, traditional and mindfulness-based, and sex therapy.
- Internists, gynecologists, and other physicians can familiarize themselves with the current understanding of an incentive-based sex response cycle to explain the logic of the woman's sexual dysfunction. Often this alone is highly therapeutic. Referral to psychologists, physicians with special interest in sexual medicine, or sex therapists may sometimes be needed.

REFERENCES

1. American Psychiatric Association. Diagnostic and statistical manual of mental disorders. 5th edition. Arlington (VA): American Psychiatric Publishing; 2013.
2. American Psychiatric Association. Diagnostic and statistical manual of mental disorders. 4th edition. Washington, DC: American Psychiatric Publishing; 2000. Text rev.
3. Brotto LA. The DSM diagnostic criteria for hypoactive sexual desire disorder in women. Arch Sex Behav 2010;39:221–39.
4. Meana M. Elucidating women's (hetero) sexual desire: definitional challenges and content expansion. J Sex Res 2010;47:104–22.
5. Toates F. An integrative theoretical framework for understanding sexual motivation, arousal, and behavior. J Sex Res 2009;46:168–93.
6. Basson R. Rethinking low sexual desire in women. BJOG 2002;109:357–63.
7. Basson R. Human sex-response cycles. J Sex Marital Ther 2001;27(1):33–43.
8. Laan E, Both S. What makes women experience desire? Fem Psychol 2008;18: 505–14.
9. Meston CM, Buss DM. Why humans have sex. Arch Sex Behav 2007;36(4): 477–507.
10. Balon R, Clayton AH. Female sexual interest/arousal disorder: a diagnosis out of thin air. Arch Sex Behav 2014;43:1227–9.
11. Balon R, Clayton AH. Further commentary on DSM-5 FSIAD diagnosis. J Sex Med 2015;12:576–7.
12. Clayton AH, DeRogatis LR, Rosen RC, et al. Intended or unintended consequences? The likely implications of raising the bar for sexual dysfunction diagnosis in the proposed DSM-V revisions: 1. For women with incomplete loss of desire or sexual receptivity. J Sex Med 2012;9:2027–39.
13. Graham CA, Brotto LA, Zucker KJ. Response to Balon and Clayton. Female sexual interest/arousal disorder is a diagnosis more on firm ground than thin air. Arch Sex Behav 2014;43:1231–4.
14. O'Loughlin JI, Basson R, Brotto LA. Women with hypoactive sexual desire disorder versus sexual interest/arousal disorder: an empirical test of raising the bar. J Sex Res 2018;55(6):734–46.
15. Hayes R, Dennerstein L. The impact of aging on sexual function and sexual dysfunction in women: a review of population-based studies. J Sex Med 2005; 2:317–30.

16. Wilcox AJ, Baird DD, Dunson DB, et al. On the frequency of intercourse around ovulation: evidence for biological influences. Hum Reprod 2004;19(7):1539–43.
17. Basson R, Brotto LA, Petkau J, et al. Role of androgens in women's sexual dysfunction. Menopause 2010;17(5):962–71.
18. Basson R, O' Loughliin JI, Weinberg J, et al. Dehydroepiandrosterone and cortisol as markers of HPA axis dysregulation in women with low sexual desire. Psychoneuroendocrinology 2019;104:259–68.
19. Wåhlin-Jacobsen S, Pedersen AT, Kristensen E, et al. Is there a correlation between androgens and sexual desire in women? J Sex Med 2015;12:358–73.
20. Wåhlin-Jacobsen S, Kristensen E, Pedersen AT, et al. Androgens and psychosocial factors related to sexual dysfunctions in premenopausal women. J Sex Med 2017;14:366–79.
21. Zheng J, Islam RM, Skiba M, et al. Associations between androgens and sexual function in premenopausal women: a cross-sectional study. Lancet Diabetes 2020;8(8):693–702.
22. Islam RM, Bell RJ, Green S, et al. Safety and efficacy of testosterone for women: a systematic review and meta-analysis of randomised controlled trial data. Lancet Diabetes Endocrinol 2019;10:754–66.
23. Snabes M, Zborowski J, Simes S. Libigel does not differentiate from placebo therapy in the treatment of hypoactive sexual desire in postmenopausal women. J Sex Med 2012;9(suppl 3):171.
24. McCabe MP, Sharlip ID, Lewis R, et al. Incidence and prevalence of sexual dysfunction in women and men: a consensus statement from the Fourth International Consultation on Sexual Medicine 2015. J Sex Med 2016;13:144–52.
25. Avis NE. Sexual function and aging in men and women: community and population-based studies. J Gend Specif Med 2000;3:37–41.
26. Geist SH, Salmon UJ, Gaines JA, et al. The biologic effects of androgen (testosterone propionate) in women. JAMA 1940;114(16):1539–44.
27. Capelletti M, Wallen K. Increasing women's sexual desire: the comparative effectiveness of estrogens and androgens. Horm Behav 2016;78:178–93.
28. Labrie F, Belangér A, Belangér P, et al. Androgen glucuronides, instead of testosterone, as the new markers of androgenic activity in women. J Steroid Biochem Mol Biol 2006;99:182–8.
29. Korkidakis K, Reid R. Testosterone in women: measurement and therapeutic use. J Obstet Gynecol Can 2017;39(3):124–30.
30. Aziz A, Brannstrom M, Bergquist C, et al. Perimenopausal androgen decline after oophorectomy does not influence sexuality or psychological well-being. Fertil Steril 2005;83:1021–8.
31. West SL, D'Aloisio AA, Agans RP, et al. Prevalence of low sexual desire and hypoactive sexual desire disorder in a nationally representative sample of US women. Arch Intern Med 2008;168:1441–9.
32. Erekson EA, Martin DK, Zhu K, et al. Sexual function in older women after oophorectomy. Obstet Gynecol 2012;120(4):833–42.
33. Krysiak R, Drosdzol-Cop A, Skrzypulec-Plinta V, et al. Sexual function and depressive symptoms in young women with nonclassic congenital adrenal hyperplasia. J Sex Med 2016;13:34–9.
34. Roney JR, Simmons ZL. Hormonal predictors of sexual motivation in natural menstrual cycles. Horm Behav 2013;63(4):636–45.
35. van Lunsen RHW, Zimmerman Y, Coelingh Bennink HJT, et al. Maintaining physiologic testosterone levels during combined oral contraceptives by adding

dehydroepiandrosterone: II. Effects on sexual function. A phase II randomized, double-blind, placebo-controlled study. Contraception 2018;98:56–62.

36. Zimmerman Y, Foidart JM, Pintiaux A, et al. Restoring testosterone levels by adding dehydroepiandrosterone to a drospirenone containing combined oral contraceptive: II. Clinical effects. Contraception 2015;91:134–42.

37. Elraiyah T, Sonbol MB, Wang Z, et al. Clinical review: the benefits and harms of systemic testosterone therapy in postmenopausal women with normal adrenal function: a systematic review and meta-analysis. J Clin Endocrinol Metab 2014; 99(10):3543–50.

38. Jayasena CN, Alkaabi1 FM, Liebers CS, et al. Systematic review of randomized controlled trials investigating the efficacy and safety of testosterone therapy for female sexual dysfunction in postmenopausal women. Clin Endocrinol (Oxf) 2019;90:391–414.

39. Davis SR, Van Der Mooren MJ, van Lunsen RH, et al. Efficacy and safety of a testosterone patch for the treatment of hypoactive sexual desire disorder in surgically menopausal women: a randomized, placebo-controlled trial. Menopause 2006;13(3):387–96.

40. Huang G, Basaria S, Travison TG, et al. Testosterone dose-response relationships in hysterectomized women with or without oophorectomy: effects on sexual function, body composition, muscle performance and physical function in a randomized trial. Menopause 2014;21(6):612–23.

41. Sherwin BB, Gelfand MM, Brender W. Androgen enhances sexual motivation in females: a prospective, crossover study of sex steroid administration in the surgical menopause. Psychosom Med 1985;47(4):339–51.

42. Davis SR, Moreau M, Kroll R, et al. Testosterone for low libido in postmenopausal women not taking estrogen. N Engl J Med 2008;359(19):2005–17.

43. Davis SR, Davison SL, Donath S, et al. Circulating androgen levels and self-reported sexual function in women. JAMA 2005;294(1):91–6.

44. Wisniewski AB, Migeon CJ, Meyer-Bahlburg HF, et al. Complete androgen insensitivity syndrome: long-term medical, surgical, and psychosexual outcome. J Clin Endo Metab 2000;85(8):2664–9.

45. Kowalczyk R, Skrzypulec-Plinta V, Nowosielski K, et al. Sexuality in women with polycystic ovary syndrome. Ginekol Pol 2015;86:100.

46. Amiri FN, Tehrani FR, Esmailzadeh S, et al. Sexual function in women with polycystic ovary syndrome and their hormonal and clinical correlations. Int J Impot Res 2018;30(2):54–61.

47. Alexander JL, Kotz K, Dennerstein L, et al. The effects of postmenopausal hormone therapies on female sexual functioning: a review of double-blind, randomized controlled trials. Menopause 2004;11(6 Part 2 of 2):749–65.

48. Buster JE, Kingsberg SA, Aguirre O, et al. Testosterone patch for low sexual desire in surgically menopausal women: a randomized trial. Obstet Gynecol 2005;105(5 Part 1):944–52.

49. Braunstein GD, Sundwall DA, Katz M, et al. Safety and efficacy of a testosterone patch for the treatment of hypoactive sexual desire disorder in surgically menopausal women: a randomized, placebo-controlled trial. Arch Intern Med 2005; 165(14):1582.

50. Pretorius E, Arlt W, Storbeck KH. A new dawn for androgens: novel lessons from 11-oxygenated C19 steroids. Mol Cell Endocrinol 2017;441:76–85.

51. Birnbaum W, Marshall L, Werner R, et al. Oestrogen versus androgen in hormone-replacement therapy for complete androgen insensitivity syndrome: a

multicentre, randomised, placebo-controlled, double-blind crossover trial. Lancet Diabetes Endocrinol 2018;6(10):771–80.

52. Sutter B, Fehr M, Hartmann C, et al. Androgen receptor gene polymorphism and sexual function in midlife women. Arch Gynecol Obstet 2019;299(4):1173–83.

53. Wang F, Pan J, Liu Y, et al. Alternative splicing of the androgen receptor in polycystic ovary syndrome. Proc Natl Acad Sci U S A 2015;112:4743–9.

54. Ratner MH, Kumaresan V, Farb DH. Neurosteroid actions in memory and neurologic/neuropsychiatric disorders. Front Endocrinol (Lausanne) 2019;10:169.

55. Labrie F, Derogatis L, Archer D, et al. Effect of intravaginal prasterone on sexual dysfunction in postmenopausal women with vulvovaginal atrophy. J Sex Med 2015;12:2401–12.

56. Laumann EO, Das A, Waite LJ. Sexual dysfunction among older adults: prevalence and risk factors from a nationally representative U.S. probability sample of men and women. J Sex Med 2008;5:2300–11.

57. Dennerstein L, Guthrie JR, Hayes RD, et al. Sexual function, dysfunction, and sexual distress in a prospective, population-based sample of mid-aged Australian-born women. J Sex Med 2008;5:2291–9.

58. Mitchell KR, Mercer CH, Ploubidis GB, et al. Sexual function in Britain: findings from the third National Survey of Sexual Attitudes and Lifestyles (NATSAL-3). Lancet 2013;382:1817–29.

59. Basson R. Sexual function of women with chronic illness and cancer. Womens Health (Lond) 2010;6(3):407–29.

60. Chadwick SB, Burke SM, Goldey KL, et al. Sexual desire in sexual minority and majority women and men: the multifaceted sexual desire questionnaire. Arch Sex Behav 2017;46(8):2465–84.

61. Basson R, Schultz WW. Sexual sequelae of general medical disorders. Lancet 2007;369:409–24.

62. Basson R. The female sexual response: the role of drugs in the management of sexual dysfunction. Obstet Gynecol 2001;98:350–2.

63. Both S, Everaerd W, Laan E. Desire emerges from excitement: a psychophysiological perspective on sexual motivation. In: Janssen E, editor. The psychophysiology of sex. Bloomington (IN): Indiana University Press; 2007. p. 327–39.

64. Nelson AL, Purdon C. Non-erotic thoughts, attentional focus, and sexual problems in a community sample. Arch Sex Behav 2011;40(2):395–406.

65. Nobre PJ, Pinto-Gouveia J. Cognitions, emotions, and sexual response: analysis of the relationship among automatic thoughts, emotional responses, and sexual arousal. Arch Sex Behav 2008;37(4):652–61.

66. Basson R, Bronner G. Management and rehabilitation of neurological patients with sexual dysfunction. neurology of sexual and bladder disorders. Handbook Neurol 2015;130:414–34.

67. Brotto LA, Basson R. Group mindfulness-based therapy significantly improves sexual desire in women. Behav Res Ther 2014;57:43–54.

68. Stephenson KR. Mindfulness-based therapies for sexual dysfunction: a review of potential theory-based mechanisms of change. Mindfulness 2017;8:527–43.

Risks of Testosterone for Postmenopausal Women

JoAnn V. Pinkerton, MD, NCMP[a],*, Isabella Blackman, BA[a],
Edward Alexander Conner, MD[a], Andrew M. Kaunitz, MD, NCMP[b]

KEYWORDS

- Androgen • Testosterone • Risks • Safety • Menopause • Women
- Hypoactive sexual desire disorder • Genitourinary syndrome of menopause

KEY POINTS

- For healthy postmenopausal women with hypoactive sexual desire disorder (HSDD) not due to other correctable reasons, transdermal testosterone therapy, dosed within the premenopausal physiologic range, improves sexual desire, sexually satisfying acts, and decreases sexual distress in menopausal women in trials up to 24 months.
- The decision to use testosterone therapy for the treatment of HSDD requires balancing the benefits on sexual desire, with the lack of available government-approved transdermal testosterone therapy for women and lack of long-term safety data for cardiovascular, cancer, and cognitive risks.
- Major adverse events reported with transdermal testosterone include hair growth and acne. Virilization, voice deepening, and clitoromegaly are rare. No negative impact on mood, cognition, or cardiovascular events has been reported. Transdermal therapy is preferred, as oral testosterone is associated with decreased serum high-density lipoprotein concentrations. Long-term consequences of the relatively high serum testosterone concentrations found with supraphysiologic dosing, such as pellets or injections, are unknown.
- No adverse effects on breast cancer or mammographic breast density have been seen with use of testosterone, but data are limited. Abnormal uterine bleeding has been reported, but no increased risk of endometrial hyperplasia or cancer.
- Discussions about treating HSDD with "off-label" testosterone includes counseling about risks and uncertainties of treatment and adverse events. Pretreatment testosterone levels and monitoring levels on therapy to avoid supraphysiologic dosing is recommended. If no benefit is seen by 6 months, discontinuation is recommended.

[a] Department of Obstetrics and Gynecology, Division of Midlife Health, University of Virginia Health System, Midlife Health Center University of Virginia Health System, PO Box 801104, Charlottesville, VA 22908, USA; [b] University of Florida College of Medicine Jacksonville, UF Health Women's Specialists, Building 2, Suite 20, 4549 Emerson Street, Jacksonville, FL 32207, USA
* Corresponding author. Department of Obstetrics and Gynecology, Division of Midlife Health, University of Virginia Health System, Midlife Health Center University of Virginia Health System, PO Box 801104, Charlottesville, VA 22908.
E-mail address: jvp9u@virginia.edu
Twitter: jvp9u1 (J.V.P.)

Endocrinol Metab Clin N Am 50 (2021) 139–150
https://doi.org/10.1016/j.ecl.2020.10.007
0889-8529/21/© 2020 Elsevier Inc. All rights reserved.
endo.theclinics.com

INTRODUCTION

Androgen levels vary with age, with steep declines in the early reproductive years and after surgical menopause, but with minimal variation during natural menopause transition.[1] The postmenopausal ovary seems to be a site of ongoing testosterone production, with small increases in later years.[1] Hypoactive sexual desire disorder (HSDD) consists of an absence of sexual fantasies and desire for sexual activity.[2] Randomized clinical trial (RCT) evidence supports the use of transdermal testosterone therapy, either alone or in combination with menopausal hormone therapy (MHT), dosed to result in premenopausal physiologic testosterone concentrations, for women with HSDD after either natural or surgical menopause.[3] Multiple, double-blind, placebo-controlled RCTs of a transdermal testosterone, 300 mcg/d, patch in women (n>2269)[4] with natural or surgical menopause showed meaningful improvements in female sexual desire, with on average one additional satisfying sexual episode per month, improvement in desire, arousal, orgasm, pleasure, and responsiveness, along with a reduction in sexually related distress.[5–7]

Despite phase III trials supporting the efficacy and safety of transdermal testosterone therapy in treating HSDD in menopausal women, long-term safety data assessing cardiovascular, cancer, and cognitive outcome are lacking. Concerns about lack of long-term safety data, along with skepticism regarding the clinical meaningfulness of the improvement in sexually satisfying acts of one per month, led the Federal Drug Administration (FDA) in 2004 to deny approval of a 300 mcg patch for the treatment of HSDD.[8] This testosterone patch was licensed by the European Medicines Agency for HSDD in women with surgically induced menopause on concomitant estrogen therapy, but marketing was discontinued in 2012 due to inadequate commercial sales. A second product, once daily transdermal hydroalcoholic testosterone gel, 300 mcg, applied daily to the upper arm skin, increased serum-free testosterone levels in postmenopausal women to the physiologic premenopausal range. Development was discontinued despite decreased sexual distress due to lack of significant improvement over placebo in number of days with sexually satisfying events and no increase in mean sexual desire.[9] Despite FDA-approved products for testosterone replacement therapy in men, no FDA-approved products for women are currently marketed. In Western Australia, a state-approved 1% transdermal testosterone pharmaceutical grade cream is available.

Before considering testosterone therapy for women with HSDD, clinicians should address relationship issues, medications, depression or other mood disorders, as well as genitourinary syndrome of menopause (GSM). Clinicians should be aware that the findings regarding transdermal testosterone do not apply to compounded non-FDA approved testosterone creams, reduced dosages of male-approved products for hypogonadism, pellets, testosterone injections, or other formulations resulting in uncertain dosing or supraphysiologic levels of testosterone.[3,6]

Testosterone Adverse Events in Postmenopausal Women

In RCTs conducted in postmenopausal women, safety data for the 300 mcg testosterone patch, dosed in the premenopausal physiologic range, have been reassuring. The most common adverse events included patch location site reactions, acne, breast tenderness, headache, and hair growth.[10] No significant changes from baseline or among treatment groups were seen for liver function, blood counts, lipid profiles, clotting measures, or carbohydrate metabolism.[3,6,10,11] In contrast with transdermal testosterone, serum high-density lipoprotein (HDL) cholesterol levels decline slightly in postmenopausal women receiving oral testosterone, with unknown impact on cardiovascular risk. Hirsutism and acne are dose and duration dependent and usually reversible. Higher testosterone levels have been associated with rare virilizing changes, clitoromegaly, and deepening of the voice, thought to be irreversible.[6]

Because clinical trials have not exceeded 2 years duration, the long-term safety of testosterone with respect to cardiovascular outcomes, breast or uterine cancer, and cognition in postmenopausal women is unknown.[6] Similarly, safety data for premenopausal women are lacking.

Testosterone and Risks of Cardiovascular Disease

Based on higher risks of cardiovascular disease (CVD) in men compared with women and a higher risk of cardiometabolic disease in women with androgen excess such as polycystic ovarian syndrome, concern exists that androgens are atherogenic in women.[12] Epidemiologic studies suggest endogenous free testosterone is associated with an increased risk of CVD.[6,12] Experts speculate impaired insulin sensitivity (polycystic ovary syndrome) and lowered sex hormone binding globulin levels (SHBG) are responsible for this elevated risk.[12–16] Administration of oral testosterone and dehydroepiandrosterone (DHEA) cause undesirable effects on HDL-cholesterol and low-density lipoprotein (LDL)-cholesterol levels.[17] Short-term (12–24 months) RCTs of transdermal and injectable testosterone have not shown adverse effects on lipids or heart disease *"in doses that approximate physiologic testosterone concentrations for premenopausal women,"* (equivalent 300 mcg/d).[3]

Testosterone therapy has not been associated with increased blood pressure, blood glucose, or HbA1c levels in trials up to 24 months.[3] Most studies included women using menopausal hormone therapy, making it difficult to interpret the effects of testosterone alone on the nonsignificant trend of increased risk of venous thrombosis. RCTs of testosterone therapy for HSDD have excluded women at high risk of cardiometabolic disease. No information is available about effect of testosterone supplementation on large elastic arterial stiffening.[17] A small 6-month RCT of transdermal patch in older women with heart failure found improved functional capacity, insulin resistance, and muscle strength but has not been replicated.[18]

The absence of cardiovascular (CV) risk with physiologic testosterone dosing in low-risk women up to 24 months does not provide evidence to support the use of testosterone for prevention or treatment of CVD. Existing data do not provide evidence for the safety of testosterone in women at elevated risk of CVD, use of supraphysiologic doses, or longer term therapy.[3]

Testosterone and Risk of Breast Cancer

The role of androgens in the genesis of breast cancer is complex, and data are limited. Sixty to eighty percent of breast cancers express androgen receptors.[19] Breast cancer proliferation is stimulated by testosterone and its metabolite dihydrotestosterone and inhibited by androgen receptor antagonists.[20–22] Some studies suggest exogenous androgens increase risk of breast cancer,[23] whereas some preclinical and clinical trials suggest decreased risk due to antiproliferative effects of testosterone in the breast.[24,25]

Esterified estrogen-methyltestosterone therapy in the Women's Health Initiative observational study was not associated with an excess risk of breast cancer (hazard ratio 1.06, 95% confidence interval 0.82 to 1.36).[26] Review of data from RCTs[3] and a systemic review[25] found short-term transdermal testosterone therapy, dosed to achieve premenopausal physiologic range, did not increase breast cancer incidence. In a 52-week trial of 279 menopausal women using transdermal testosterone not on menopausal hormone therapy, changes in mammographic breast density from baseline were small and similar in the testosterone and placebo groups.[7,27]

Similarly, a small RCT of 99 postmenopausal women on continuous combined estradiol 2 mg/norethindrone acetate 1 mg, randomized to a 300 mcg/d testosterone patch or placebo showed similar change in breast density at 6 months as placebo.[28] Fine-needle breast aspiration biopsy at baseline and after 6 months found more than 5-fold increase ($P<.001$) in total breast epithelial and stromal cell proliferation from baseline for those on estrogen/progestin plus placebo. No significant increase in the percentage of proliferating cells positively stained by the Ki-67/MIB-1 antibody, a biomarker for breast carcinoma, was found in breast tissue from participants randomized to testosterone (1.6% vs 2.0%).[29]

Observational studies have found no increased risk of breast cancer in prior testosterone users.[30] However, clinical trials lack sufficient size and duration to ascertain safety of testosterone on risk of breast cancer.[3] Adequately powered RCTs designed with a primary end point of breast cancer incidence are needed to better assess testosterone's effects on the breast. Until then, systemic androgens cannot be recommended for women with, or at high risk, for breast cancer.

Testosterone and Cancers of the Endometrium and Ovary

Androgens are synthesized in the ovary and adrenal gland. In vitro data suggest androgens do not directly stimulate the endometrium.[31] Aromatase activity converting testosterone to estrogen has been observed in endometrial cancer cells.[6] Androgen receptor–mediated effects have been studied in human and rat endometrial tissue and are being evaluated for their role in endometrial cell proliferation, during menses, and in endometriosis and endometrial cancer.[32,33] Exogenous testosterone dosed at physiologic premenopausal levels has not been independently associated with risk of endometrial hyperplasia or cancer in RCTs up to 24 months.[6] Most studies conducted in menopausal women showed either no effect or atrophic endometrium on endometrial biopsy. Bleeding was more frequent on the 300 mcg transdermal patch than on the 150 mcg (10.6% compared with 2.7%), with atrophy or insufficient tissue found on biopsy.[34]

Abnormal uterine bleeding in menopausal woman receiving testosterone should be evaluated with transvaginal ultrasound and endometrial biopsy, just as in other menopausal women. A study of 58 postmenopausal patients using combined estradiol and testosterone implants (supraphysiologic hormone levels) found 44 patients with endometrial thickening greater than 5 mm after 2 years. Polypoid lesions were seen in 61.3% of the hysteroscopy cases, a normal uterine cavity in 31.8%, and submucous myoma in the remaining 6.8%. Histology confirmed an endometrial polyp in 38.6% of cases, normal endometrium in 31.8%, simple endometrial hyperplasia in 20.4%, and myoma and atrophic endometrium in 4.5%. The investigators theorized testosterone might be antiproliferative on the background endometrium but not on polyps.[35]

Endogenous elevated androgen levels have been associated with increased risk of endometrioid and mucinous tumors and a decreased incidence of high-grade serous ovarian tumors.[36] Published data do not address the impact of supplemental (exogenous) androgens on risk of ovarian cancer.

Cognition and Mood

Cognition
The brain expresses receptors for estrogen and testosterone, particularly in regions responsible for memory and higher cognitive function.[37] In the decade preceding menopause, the midcycle surge of free testosterone and androstenedione is lost.[38]

If physiologic concentrations of androgens influence cognitive performance in women, a decrease in testosterone production with normal adrenal aging and menopause could be associated with cognitive changes in older women. Observational studies find men tend to perform better in visuospatial tasks and women have better verbal memory, suggesting sex hormones exert sexually dimorphic effects on cognitive domains.[39] Observational data suggest for older women, not selected for optimal health, endogenous testosterone levels have a negative association with verbal memory.[40]

Some studies suggest supplemental testosterone or adding testosterone to estrogen treatment might improve cognition, including memory. Tests of memory and logical reasoning improved in surgically oophorectomized women following 2 months of testosterone treatment.[41] One RCT of physiologically dosed transdermal testosterone, adjusted for age and baseline score, found verbal learning and memory significantly improved at week 26 compared with placebo. No other cognitive domains benefitted from testosterone nor was general psychological well-being improved.[42] A meta-analysis of RCTs found no increase in memory with testosterone with tests of immediate and delayed recall or measures of cognitive performance.[7]

The statistically significant improvements in verbal memory seen with physiologically dosed testosterone therapy in studies of postmenopausal women underscore the need for further investigation of testosterone's impact on cognition in postmenopausal women. Current evidence does not support use of testosterone for prevention or treatment of cognitive decline in this population.[3]

Mood

Transdermal testosterone cream (10 mg) daily in a small cross-over RCT of 36 hysterectomized women receiving estrogen significantly improved sexual desire, frequency of sex, receptivity, and initiation without improvement in mood, energy, lipids, blood pressure, or weight.[43] A 24-week RCT of 300 mcg testosterone patch in 77 surgically menopausal women found significantly reduced personal distress compared with placebo, with only a trend (borderline difference) for positive well-being domain and general health domains.[44] A 12-week RCT of 44 women (35–55 years) on stable doses of antidepressants (selective serotonin reuptake inhibitors/serotonin and norepinephrine reuptake inhibitors) with treatment-emergent loss of libido received 300 mcg/d testosterone or placebo patch. Transdermal testosterone led to a significant increase in number of sexually satisfying events versus placebo but no overall improvement in sexual satisfaction scores or well-being. These data suggest physiologic transdermal testosterone may have a role in antidepressant emergent loss of libido, if changing dose or type of antidepressant is unsuccessful.[45] No treatment benefit or worsening was found for general well-being, mood, or depression.[3] Testosterone showed improvement in well-being for premenopausal not postmenopausal women; however data are inconclusive.[46,47]

Testosterone and Musculoskeletal System

Low serum androgen concentrations are associated with lower bone mineral density (BMD) and an increase in fracture risk in some studies. RCTs testing the benefit of adding testosterone to estrogen replacement therapy found no significant increase in BMD.[48,49] No data on the benefits or risks of androgen supplementation are available for women with osteoporosis. No significant effect of testosterone administered in physiologic doses was found on lean body mass, total body fat, or muscle strength,[3,50,51] although benefit was seen in higher doses with higher serum levels.[46]

Androgens and the Lower Genital Tract

The clitoris, vestibule, vestibular glands, urethra, anterior vaginal wall, periurethral tissue, and pelvic floor are androgen responsive. Limited data suggest systemic testosterone treatment improves vaginal epithelial health and blood flow.[52]

Vaginal testosterone therapy tested in small short-term open-label trials has been studied as a treatment of GSM, with improvement in vaginal cytology, vaginal pH, and improved dyspareunia in women with breast cancer. Improvement in dyspareunia without estrogenic effects on vagina were found in a small RCT with vaginal testosterone 300 mcg/d for women on aromatase inhibitors; no systemic testosterone absorption was seen.[53]

Higher doses of intravaginal testosterone (5000 μg 3 times/wk) in women on aromatase inhibitors resulted in higher serum levels, without improving sexual satisfaction, and potentially increasing side effects of hair growth or acne.[54]

Intravaginal DHEA, a prohormone converted by vaginal epithelial cells into estrogen and testosterone, is FDA-approved for dyspareunia due to GSM[55] and is being studied for HSDD. Serum steroid concentrations were found to be within normal postmenopausal values in women after 12 weeks of use.[56]

No published data on safety and efficacy in breast cancer survivors on aromatase inhibitors are available for the approved product. A compounded vaginal DHEA was associated with increased estradiol, *DHEA-S*, and testosterone levels, within lower quartile of normal postmenopausal levels, which was dose—dependent. No increase in estradiol levels was found for those on an aromatase inhibitor.[57]

"OFF-LABEL" TESTOSTERONE FOR HYPOACTIVE SEXUAL DESIRE DISORDER FOR POSTMENOPAUSAL WOMEN

In the absence of FDA-approved transdermal testosterone therapy for HSDD for postmenopausal women, major medical societies remain concerned about risks of compounding therapies, using fractional doses of male formulations and supraphysiologic dosing of hormones. Adequately powered RCTS are not available to show safety or efficacy of compounded testosterone for any indication, including improvement of HSDD. Off-label testosterone therapy has been used as a compounded topical cream testosterone ointment or cream (1%), 0.5 g daily, applied topically to the arms, thighs, or lower abdomen. A reduced dose of a testosterone gel (1%) FDA approved for men (eg, AndroGel, Testim) prescribed at one-tenth of standard dose for male hypogonadism should result in physiologic premenopausal serum levels.[58] If off-label testosterone is considered for HSDD, a prudent strategy is outlined in **Box 1** to ensure the patients are well counseled about potential risks and lack of safety and efficacy data.

DISCUSSION

For reproductive-age women, low testosterone is unlikely to be a primary issue and androgen therapy is rarely a consideration. Data are limited for efficacy or safety, with concern about inadvertent developing fetus exposure leading to masculinization.

Despite some data on endogenous testosterone and health effects, the primary reason to consider supplemental testosterone in postmenopausal women is HSDD. Efficacy and short-term safety have been shown for transdermal testosterone dosed within physiologic premenopausal levels.

Unfortunately, despite data showing effectiveness and safety, there are no FDA-approved transdermal testosterone products for women. Compounded testosterone

---

Box 1
Counseling strategy for "off-label" testosterone for postmenopausal hypoactive sexual desire disorder

Informed consent should be documented and address the following:
- Off-label FDA-nonapproved status
- Goal to keep total testosterone levels within premenopausal physiologic range
- Modest efficacy
- Potential androgenic effects (hair growth, acne, virilization)
- Lack of long-term safety data regarding breast and endometrial cancer, CVD, and cognition
- Need for monitoring serum total testosterone levels and for adverse events
- Discontinuation if no benefit noted at 3 to 6 months

Concerns about compounding testosterone
- Potential of over- or underdosing, contaminants, and sterility issues
- Lack of RCT data on safety and efficacy
- Lack of a label
- Lack of FDA approval and monitoring
- Potential transference of compounded cream/gel to pets or people

Supraphysiologic levels may result when testosterone products formulated and approved specifically for men are used in women, even when dosed appropriately using fractional doses (one-tenth)

Supraphysiologic dosing of testosterone with pellets or injections is not recommended due to concerns of higher systemic levels and potential risks

Measurement of serum total testosterone levels, before treatment and episodically is to maintain serum levels within premenopausal physiologic range

---

therapy cannot be recommended for the treatment of HSDD unless an approved equivalent preparation is not available and then only considered for well-counseled women (see **Box 1**). Safety or efficacy data are lacking for compounded testosterone products, reduced doses of male-approved therapies, or supraphysiologic dosing with pellets and injections, with concern about potential CV risks, breast or uterine cancers, and unknown effects on cognition. Developing safe and effective transdermal testosterone therapies, dosed to achieve serum levels within premenopausal physiologic ranges, represents an unmet need for postmenopausal women with HSDD, with longer-term studies needed to assess risks of CV, cancer, and cognitive outcomes.

SUMMARY

Although transdermal testosterone, dosed within the premenopausal physiologic range, has been shown to be safe and effective for postmenopausal women with HSDD after other contributors have been addressed (relationship and psychosocial issues, medications, GSM), there are no FDA-approved testosterone formulations for women, primarily due to lack of consistent efficacy data and a lack of long-term data regarding efficacy and safety.

Transdermal administration of testosterone has the advantages of avoiding the potential hepatic toxicity of oral androgens, is easily discontinued, and allows more physiologic control of testosterone levels than subcutaneous implants, while maintaining serum testosterone levels within the normal premenopausal range. Adverse events are usually mild and include hirsutism, acne, and hair loss. Systemic oral or supraphysiologic dosing raises concern about potential CV, thrombotic, and cancer risks. Women with HSDD who are candidates for physiologically dosed transdermal therapy should be counseled regarding the lack of FDA-approved formulations, concerns about nonapproved testosterone therapy, and the lack of long-term safety data (see **Box 1**).

Both intravaginal DHEA suppositories and intravaginal testosterone need further study for effectiveness for sexual concerns, particularly among breast cancer survivors on aromatase inhibitors.

CLINICS CARE POINTS

- Candidates for testosterone treatment are postmenopausal women with decreased sexual desire associated with personal distress after other identifiable causes are evaluated (physical and psychosocial factors, medications).
- Evaluation includes subjective assessments of sexual response, desire, and satisfaction and monitoring for potential adverse androgenic effects of therapy (hair growth, acne).
- Routine measurement of testosterone is not recommended, as no testosterone level has been clearly linked to a clinical syndrome of hypoandrogenism or androgen insufficiency in women.
- Contraindications to testosterone therapy include women with breast or uterine cancer or with cardiovascular or liver disease.
- Transdermal therapies are preferred over oral to avoid first-pass hepatic effects and negative effects on HDL and LDL
- Adverse events, primarily seen with oral or higher doses of testosterone, include hirsutism, deepening of voice, and changes in coagulation profile, hematocrit, or mood.
- If "off-label" testosterone is used, laboratory testing of testosterone levels is recommended to monitor for supraphysiologic levels before and during therapy, not to diagnose testosterone insufficiency.
- There are no available government-approved transdermal testosterone products for postmenopausal women in the United States and no consistent ways to prescribe physiologic testosterone for women (see **Box 1**).
- Counseling regarding the lack of long-term safety data for breast and uterine cancer, stroke, CVD, thrombosis, and cognition; possible androgenic side effects; lack of government-approved therapies for women; and potential benefits on sexual desire should be provided and documented before initiating "off-label" therapy. Discontinue testosterone if continued benefit is not seen after 3 to 6 months.
- Large, longer-term RCTs are needed to address safety concerns.

DISCLOSURE

J.V. Pinkerton—none in past 24 months. I. Blackman—no disclosures. E.A. Conner—no disclosures. A.M. Kaunitz: Advisory Boards: Mithra, Pfizer; Clinical trials (financial support to University of Florida): Mithra.

REFERENCES

1. Davison SL, Bell R, Donath S, et al. Androgen levels in adult females: changes with age, menopause, and oophorectomy. J Clin Endocrinol Metab 2005;90(7):3847–53.

2. Kingsberg SA. The hypoactive sexual desire disorder registry to characterize the natural history and outcomes of women with hypoactive sexual desire disorder. Menopause 2012;19(4):379–81.
3. Davis SR, Baber R, Panay N, et al. Global consensus position statement on the use of testosterone therapy for women. J Clin Endocrinol Metab 2019;104(10): 4660–6.
4. Ganesan K, Habboush Y, Sultan S. Transdermal testosterone in female hypoactive sexual desire disorder: a rapid qualitative systematic review using grading of recommendations assessment, development and evaluation. Cureus 2018; 10(3):e2401.
5. Davis SR, Worsley R, Miller KK, et al. Androgens and female sexual function and dysfunction–findings from the fourth international consultation of sexual medicine. J Sex Med 2016;13(2):168–78.
6. Wierman ME, Arlt W, Basson R, et al. Androgen therapy in women: a reappraisal: an endocrine Society clinical practice guideline. J Clin Endocrinol Metab 2014; 99(10):3489–510.
7. Islam RM, Bell RJ, Green S, et al. Safety and efficacy of testosterone for women: a systematic review and meta-analysis of randomised controlled trial data. Lancet Diabetes Endocrinol 2019;7(10):754–66.
8. FDA. FDA intrinsa advisory committee background docuent overview. 2004. Available at: https://wayback.archive-it.org/7993/20170405114627/https://www.fda.gov/ohrms/dockets/ac/04/briefing/2004-4082B1_02_A-FDA-Intrinsa-Overview.htm. Accessed May 2, 2020.
9. Waldman T, Shufelt C, Braunstein G. Safety and efficacy of transdermal testosterone for treatment of hypoactive sexual desire disorder. Clin Investig 2012; 2(4):423–32.
10. Clayton AH, Goldstein I, Kim NN, et al. The international society for the study of women's sexual health process of care for management of hypoactive sexual desire disorder in women. Mayo Clin Proc 2018;93(4):467–87.
11. Achilli C, Pundir J, Ramanathan P, et al. Efficacy and safety of transdermal testosterone in postmenopausal women with hypoactive sexual desire disorder: a systematic review and meta-analysis. Fertil Steril 2017;107(2):475–82.e15.
12. Lo JC, Feigenbaum SL, Yang J, et al. Epidemiology and adverse cardiovascular risk profile of diagnosed polycystic ovary syndrome. J Clin Endocrinol Metab 2006;91(4):1357–63.
13. Legro RS, Kunselman AR, Dunaif A. Prevalence and predictors of dyslipidemia in women with polycystic ovary syndrome. Am J Med 2001;111(8):607–13.
14. Berneis K, Rizzo M, Lazzarini V, et al. Atherogenic lipoprotein phenotype and low-density lipoproteins size and subclasses in women with polycystic ovary syndrome. J Clin Endocrinol Metab 2007;92(1):186–9.
15. Barrett-Connor E, Goodman-Gruen D. Prospective study of endogenous sex hormones and fatal cardiovascular disease in postmenopausal women. BMJ 1995; 311(7014):1193–6.
16. Laughlin GA, Goodell V, Barrett-Connor E. Extremes of endogenous testosterone are associated with increased risk of incident coronary events in older women. J Clin Endocrinol Metab 2010;95(2):740–7.
17. Moreau KL, Babcock MC, Hildreth KL. Sex differences in vascular aging in response to testosterone. Biol Sex Differ 2020;11(1):18.
18. Iellamo F, Volterrani M, Caminiti G, et al. Testosterone therapy in women with chronic heart failure: a pilot double blind, randomized, placebo-controlled study. J Am Coll Cardiol 2010;56(16):1310–6.

19. Hu R, Dawood S, Holmes MD, et al. Androgen receptor expression and breast cancer survival in postmenopausal women. Clin Cancer Res 2011;17(7):1867–74.

20. Zhu A, Li Y, Song W, et al. Antiproliferative effect of androgen receptor inhibition in mesenchymal stem-like triple-negative breast cancer. Cell Physiol Biochem 2016; 38(3):1003–14.

21. Rampurwala M, Wisinski KB, O'Regan R. Role of the androgen receptor in triple-negative breast cancer. Clin Adv Hematol Oncol 2016;14(3):186–93.

22. Davis SR, Baber R, Panay N, et al. Response to letter to the editor: "global consensus position statement on the use of testosterone therapy for women.". J Clin Endocrinol Metab 2020;105(6):dgaa126.

23. Brusselaers N, Tamimi RM, Konings P, et al. Different menopausal hormone regimens and risk of breast cancer. Ann Oncol 2018;29(8):1771-1776.

24. Labrie F, Luu-The V, Labrie C, et al. Endocrine and intracrine sources of androgens in women: inhibition of breast cancer and other roles of androgens and their precursor dehydroepiandrosterone. Endocr Rev. 2003;24(2):152-182Gera R, Tayeh S, Chehade HE, Mokbel K. Does transdermal testosterone increase the risk of developing breast cancer? A systematic review. Anticancer Res 2018; 38(12):6615–20.

25. Gera R, Tayeh S, Chehade HE, et al. Does transdermal testosterone increase the risk of developing breast cancer? A systematic review. Anticancer Res 2018; 38(12):6615-6620.

26. Kabat GC, Kamensky V, Heo M, et al. Combined conjugated esterified estrogen plus methyltestosterone supplementation and risk of breast cancer in postmenopausal women. Maturitas 2014;79(1):70–6.

27. Davis SR, Hirschberg AL, Wagner LK, et al. The effect of transdermal testosterone on mammographic density in postmenopausal women not receiving systemic estrogen therapy. J Clin Endocrinol Metab 2009;94(12):4907–13.

28. Hofling M, Lundstrom E, Azavedo E, et al. Testosterone addition during menopausal hormone therapy: effects on mammographic breast density. Climacteric 2007;10(2):155–63.

29. Hofling M, Hirschberg AL, Skoog L, et al. Testosterone inhibits estrogen/progestogen-induced breast cell proliferation in postmenopausal women. Menopause 2007;14(2):183–90.

30. Davis SR. Cardiovascular and cancer safety of testosterone in women. Curr Opin Endocrinol Diabetes Obes 2011;18(3):198–203.

31. Zang H, Sahlin L, Masironi B, et al. Effects of testosterone and estrogen treatment on the distribution of sex hormone receptors in the endometrium of postmenopausal women. Menopause 2008;15(2):233–9.

32. Gibson DA, Simitsidellis I, Collins F, et al. Endometrial Intracrinology: oestrogens, androgens and endometrial disorders. Int J Mol Sci 2018;19(10):3276.

33. Simitsidellis I, Saunders PTK, Gibson DA. Androgens and endometrium: new insights and new targets. Mol Cell Endocrinol 2018;465:48–60.

34. Davis SR, Moreau M, Kroll R, et al. Testosterone for low libido in postmenopausal women not taking estrogen. N Engl J Med 2008;359(19):2005–17.

35. Filho AM, Barbosa IC, Maia H Jr, et al. Effects of subdermal implants of estradiol and testosterone on the endometrium of postmenopausal women. Gynecol Endocrinol 2007;23(9):511–7.

36. Ose J, Poole EM, Schock H, et al. Androgens are differentially associated with ovarian cancer subtypes in the ovarian cancer cohort consortium. Cancer Res 2017;77(14):3951–60.

37. Huang G, Wharton W, Travison TG, et al. Effects of testosterone administration on cognitive function in hysterectomized women with low testosterone levels: a dose-response randomized trial. J Endocrinol Invest 2015;38(4):455–61.
38. Mushayandebvu T, Castracane VD, Gimpel T, et al. Evidence for diminished mid-cycle ovarian androgen production in older reproductive aged women. Fertil Steril 1996;65(4):721–3.
39. Maccoby EE, Jacklin CN. The psychology of sex differences. Stanford (CA): Stanford University Press; 1974.
40. Hogervorst E, Bandelow S. Sex steroids to maintain cognitive function in women after the menopause: a meta-analyses of treatment trials. Maturitas 2010;66(1): 56–71.
41. Sherwin BB. Estrogen and/or androgen replacement therapy and cognitive functioning in surgically menopausal women. Psychoneuroendocrinology 1988;13(4): 345–57.
42. Davis SR, Jane F, Robinson PJ, et al. Transdermal testosterone improves verbal learning and memory in postmenopausal women not on oestrogen therapy. Clin Endocrinol (Oxf) 2014;81(4):621–8.
43. El-Hage G, Eden JA, Manga RZ. A double-blind, randomized, placebo-controlled trial of the effect of testosterone cream on the sexual motivation of menopausal hysterectomized women with hypoactive sexual desire disorder. Climacteric 2007;10(4):335–43.
44. Davis SR, van der Mooren MJ, van Lunsen RH, et al. Efficacy and safety of a testosterone patch for the treatment of hypoactive sexual desire disorder in surgically menopausal women: a randomized, placebo controlled trial. Menopause 2006;13:387–96.
45. Fooladi E, Bell RJ, Jane F, et al. Testosterone improves antidepressant-emergent loss of libido in women: Findings from a randomized, double-blind, placebo-controlled trial. J Sex Med 2014;11:831–9.
46. Huang G, Basaria S, Travison TG, et al. Testosterone dose-response relationships in hysterectomized women with or without oophorectomy: effects on sexual function, body composition, muscle performance and physical function in a randomized trial. Menopause 2014;21(6):612–23.
47. Goldstat R, Briganti E, Tran J, et al. Transdermal testosterone therapy improves well-being, mood, and sexual function in premenopausal women. Menopause 2003;10(5):390–8.
48. Watts NB, Notelovitz M, Timmons MC, et al. Comparison of oral estrogens and estrogens plus androgen on bone mineral density, menopausal symptoms, and lipid-lipoprotein profiles in surgical menopause. Obstet Gynecol 1995;85(4): 529–37.
49. Vegunta S, Kling JM, Kapoor E. Androgen therapy in women. J Womens Health (Larchmt) 2020;29(1):57–64.
50. Davis SR, Walker KZ, Strauss BJ. Effects of estradiol with and without testosterone on body composition and relationships with lipids in postmenopausal women. Menopause 2000;7(6):395–401.
51. Davis SR, McCloud P, Strauss BJ, et al. Testosterone enhances estradiol's effects on postmenopausal bone density and sexuality. Maturitas 2008;61(1–2):17–26. Original work published in Maturitas. 1995;21(3):227-236.
52. Simon JA, Goldstein I, Kim NN, et al. The role of androgens in the treatment of genitourinary syndrome of menopause (GSM): International Society for the study of women's sexual health (ISSWSH) expert consensus panel review. Menopause 2018;25(7):837–47.

53. Davis SR, Robinson PJ, Jane F, et al. Intravaginal testosterone improves sexual satisfaction and vaginal symptoms associated with aromatase inhibitors. J Clin Endocrinol Metab 2018;103(11):4146–54.
54. Melisko ME, Goldman ME, Hwang J, et al. Vaginal testosterone cream vs estradiol vaginal ring for vaginal dryness or decreased libido in women receiving aromatase inhibitors for early-stage breast cancer: a randomized clinical trial. JAMA Oncol 2017;3(3):313–9.
55. Labrie F, Martel C, Berube R, et al. Intravaginal prasterone (DHEA) provides local action without clinically significant changes in serum concentrations of estrogens or androgens. J Steroid Biochem Mol Biol 2013;138:359–67.
56. Martel C, Labrie F, Archer DF, et al. other participating members of the prasterone clinical research group. Serum steroid concentrations remain within normal postmenopausal values in women receiving daily 6.5mg intravaginal prasterone for 12 weeks. J Steroid Biochem Mol Biol 2016;159:142–53.
57. Barton DL, Shuster LT, Dockter T, et al. Systemic and local effects of vaginal dehydroepiandrosterone (DHEA): NCCTG N10C1 (Alliance). Support Care Cancer 2018;26(4):1335-1343.
58. Shifren JL. Testosterone for midlife women: the hormone of desire? Menopause 2015;22(10):1147–9.

Nonclassic Congenital Adrenal Hyperplasia
What Do Endocrinologists Need to Know?

Smita Jha, MD[a,b], Adina F. Turcu, MD, MS[c,*]

KEYWORDS

- 21-Hydroxylase deficiency • Androgens • Congenital adrenal hyperplasia • Adrenal
- Adrenal cortex

KEY POINTS

- Nonclassic congenital adrenal hyperplasia (NCCAH) has an overall prevalence of 1:200 in the US population and up to 1:30 in certain ethnic groups, particularly those of Mediterranean decscent and Ashkenazi Jews.
- Patients with NCCAH do not have adrenal insufficiency and do not need hormonal replacement.
- Hormonal screening for NCCAH with 17-hydroxyprogesterone is indicated in all patients with polycystic ovarian syndrome (PCOS)-like phenotype, as the two cannot be distinguished clinically.
- The treatment of women with NCCAH who present with signs of hyperandrogenism and who are not planning pregnancy is similar to those with PCOS and includes oral contraceptives ± antiandrogen therapy. Treatment of infertility, however, starts with glucocorticoids in NCCAH women.
- Research suggests that steroid biomarkers of primarily adrenal origin, such as 11-hydroxyandrostenedione and its downstream bioactive metabolite 11-ketotestosterone, may offer guidance regarding disease control and management of nonclassic CAH.

INTRODUCTION

Congenital adrenal hyperplasia (CAH) is a group of autosomal recessive genetic defects in cortisol synthesis. The altered negative feedback of cortisol to the hypothalamus and the pituitary gland prompts corticotropin-releasing hormone and

Sources of Funding: This work was supported by the NIH Intramural Research Program and by NIDDK (grant 1K08DK109116 awarded to A.F. Turcu) and University of Michigan M-Cubed (grant U064177 awarded to A.F. Turcu).
[a] Section on Congenital Disorders, National Institutes of Health Clinical Center, Bethesda, MD 20892, USA; [b] Metabolic Diseases Branch, National Institutes of Diabetes and Digestive and Kidney Diseases, 9000 Rockville Pike, Room 9C432A, Bethesda, MD 20892, USA; [c] Division of Metabolism, Endocrinology and Diabetes, University of Michigan, 1150 West Medical Center Drive, MSRB II, 5570B, Ann Arbor, MI 48109, USA
* Corresponding author.
E-mail address: aturcu@umich.edu
Twitter: @docsmita_jha (S.J.); @adina_turcu (A.F.T.)

adrenocorticotrophic hormone (ACTH) elevations. Increased ACTH, in turn, has 2 downstream effects: (1) it overstimulates adrenal steroidogenesis, resulting in an accumulation of steroids above the enzymatic blockage; and (2) when sustained, ACTH elevation promotes adrenal gland enlargement (hence, the term CAH). A variety of mutations in one or more genes encoding enzymes essential for cortisol synthesis **(Fig. 1)** lead to a spectrum of disorders and disease severity. In general, complete or nearly complete enzymatic defects result in overt adrenal insufficiency and are conventionally referred to as "classic" CAH. In milder forms of the disease, also termed "late-onset" or "nonclassic" CAH (NCCAH), partial enzymatic defects are overcome by ACTH elevations. These patients have compensated cortisol and aldosterone production. Defects in the gene encoding 21-hydroxylase (*CYP21A2*) account for more than 95% of all cases of CAH[1] and, unless otherwise specified, the term CAH will refer to 21-hydroxylase deficiency (21OHD) throughout this article. A brief overview of rare forms of CAH is presented in **Table 1**.

Patients with classic CAH are typically diagnosed at birth or early in life, and their transition of care to adult endocrinology occurs with the diagnosis previously established. Conversely, adult endocrinologists must know when to suspect NCCAH, which

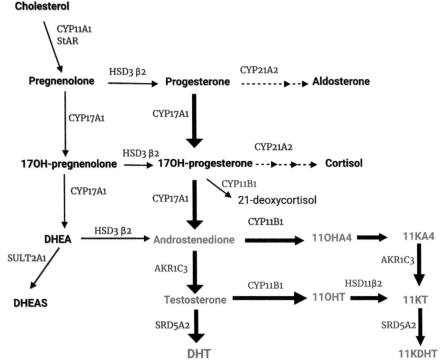

Fig. 1. Steroidogenic pathway. Genetic defects in 21-hydroxylase result in accumulation of 17OHP, which is diverted toward androgens, including: A4, T, and 11-oxygenated androgens (11OHA4 and 11OHT); the latter two are oxidized to 11KA4 and11KT, respectively, in the kidneys and other tissues. 11OHT, 11β-hydroxytestosterone; AKR1C3, 17β-hydroxysteroid dehydrogenase type 5; CYB5A, cytochrome *b*5 type A; CYP11A1, cholesterol side-chain cleavage; CYP17A1, 17α-hydroxylase/17,20-lyase; DHEA, dehydroepiandrosterone; DHEAS, dehydroepiandrosterone sulfate; HSD11B2, 11β-hydroxysteroid dehydrogenase, type 2; HSD3β2, 3β-hydroxysteroid dehydrogenase type 2; SRD5A2, steroid 5α-reductase type 2; SULT2A1, sulfotransferase 2A1.

has a considerably higher prevalence. In this review, the authors focus primarily on NCCAH.

EPIDEMIOLOGY

The worldwide incidence of classic CAH is roughly 1:14,000 to 1:18,000 births.[2] In contrast, NCCAH is relatively common, with an overall prevalence of 1:200 in the white US population,[2,3] and a higher frequency among Ashkenazi Jews, Hispanics, those of Mediterranean descent, those from the Middle East, and Eskimos.[4] Among women presenting with symptoms of androgen excess, the overall prevalence of NCCAH is approximately 4%.[5]

GENETICS OF CONGENITAL ADRENAL HYPERPLASIA

The *CYP21A2* gene is located on the long arm of chromosome 6, within the HLA locus and adjacent to the genes for the fourth component of complement,[6–8] a region within which genetic recombinations occur frequently.[9] A highly homologous nonfunctional pseudogene (*CYP21A1P*), which encodes a truncated, inactive enzyme, also resides in the vicinity.[10] Most patients with NCCAH are compound heterozygotes with different mutations in the 2 alleles.[5] Mutations that fully annul 21-hydroxylase activity, such as complete deletions, large gene conversions, and nonsense or frame-shift mutations, lead to salt-wasting CAH, in which both glucocorticoid and mineralocorticoid production is lacking. Mutations that render even minimum residual enzyme activity lead to the so-called simple virilizing CAH, whereby sufficient aldosterone synthesis occurs. In NCCAH, 20% to 60% of the enzyme activity is preserved, which ensures cortisol concentrations equal to those of unaffected individuals. NCCAH patients might harbor 1 classic and 1 nonclassic allele or 2 nonclassic alleles. Parents with NCCAH have a 1.5% to 2.5% risk of having a child with classic 21OHD.[11,12] Thus, *CYP21A2* genotyping in patients with 21OHD and their partners can refine the risk of having an affected offspring.[2]

Although a strong genotype-phenotype correlation exists for the most severe and the mildest forms of CAH, the clinical manifestations of moderate CAH forms are quite variable.[13,14] Certain mutations, such as P30L, I172N, or I2G, and combinations of mutations (homozygous vs heterozygous) can yield different phenotypes.[14] Characterizing the predominant phenotype for a given genotype can assist in genetic counseling of parents at risk of having a child with CAH.

CLINICAL FEATURES OF PATIENTS WITH CONGENITAL ADRENAL HYPERPLASIA

The clinical manifestations of CAH can result from cortisol and/or aldosterone deficiency when present (in classic CAH), and from excessive synthesis of bioactive steroids, which is prompted by ACTH and facilitated by the enzymatic blockade. In the case of 21OHD, variable degrees of androgen excess occur (see **Fig. 1**). In patients with classic 21OHD, in utero exposure to profound androgen excess leads to virilization of the genitalia in girls, which is easily identified at birth. In contrast, affected boys have minimal or no physical findings, putting them at risk for incorrect or missed diagnosis when newborn screening is not pursued. The implementation of newborn screening across all United States and several other countries has significantly decreased the death rates among infants with salt wasting 21OHD[2] and debunked the preponderance of disease in girls.

Patients with NCCAH may present during childhood with premature pubarche, which has been described as early as 6 months of age.[5] In contrast, girls with NCCAH

Table 1
Uncommon causes of congenital adrenal hyperplasia

SCC deficiency:

Prevalence:	• Rare, relatively increased prevalence in Southeastern Turkey[50] • First described in 2001
Presentation:	• Severe, early onset adrenal failure in infancy • Minimal aldosterone synthesis with high-plasma renin • 46,XY with female external genitalia but no cervix, uterus, and fallopian tubes and well-developed Wolffian duct derivatives • 46,XX have normal genitalia at birth
Diagnosis:	• Deficiency of all steroid hormones • Absent response to cosyntropin or hCG stimulation • Clinically and hormonally indistinguishable from lipoid CAH but atrophic adrenals and gonads • Genetic testing needed to differentiate lipoid CAH and SCC deficiency
Nonclassic form:	• Mutations wherein 10%–20% enzyme activity is retained • Clinically and hormonally indistinguishable from nonclassic lipoid CAH
Management:	• Physiologic replacement of GC • Supplementary salt in newborns with MC replacement thereafter • Discussion regarding orchiectomy in 46,XY patients

StAR deficiency: Lipoid CAH

Prevalence:	• Rare, with >100 patients reported • Second most common form of CAH in Korea and Japan[50]
Presentation:	• Most severe steroidogenic disorder; most present with neonatal crisis; rarely, presentations up to age 1 y[15] • Minimal aldosterone synthesis with high-plasma renin • 46,XY with female external genitalia but no cervix, uterus, and fallopian tubes but well-developed Wolffian duct derivatives, consistent with some StAR-independent T synthesis early in life • 46,XX have normal genitalia at birth and go through puberty with breast development and cyclic vaginal bleeding; anovulatory cycles as progesterone synthesis disturbed • Impaired DHEA synthesis eliminates fetoplacental estriol production
Diagnosis:	• Deficiency of all steroid hormones • Absent response to cosyntropin or hCG stimulation • Grossly enlarged adrenals • Genetic testing needed to differentiate lipoid CAH and SCC deficiency
Nonclassic form:	• Associated with mutations that retain 20%–30% activity • Mildly compromised MC secretion • Can present from toddlers to adulthood with mild adrenal insufficiency • Wide variation in gonadal function • 46,XY typically have normal-appearing external genitalia

(continued on next page)

Table 1	
(continued)	
Management:	• Physiologic replacement of GC • Supplementary salt in newborn; MC replacement thereafter • Discussion regarding orchiectomy in 46,XY patients
HSD3B2 (Δ^5-Δ^4 Isomerase) deficiency	
Prevalence:	• Very rare (<0.5% of all CAH); <1 in 1,000,000[51]
Presentation:	• Both gonads and adrenal glands affected • 46,XX may have atypical genitalia due to large amounts of DHEA, some of which is converted to T by extraadrenal HSD3B1 • 46,XY can have severe hypospadias, micropenis, bifid scrotum, and undescended testis due to inadequate T. In contrast with 21OHD, it is diagnosed earlier and more frequently in boys, and girls can remain undiagnosed
Diagnosis:	• Basal or cosyntropin-induced increase in Δ^5 steroids typically 17α-hydroxypregnenolone to $\geq$3000 ng/dL (90 nmol/L) • 17OHP can be high due to activity of extraadrenal HSD3B1 • Molecular genetic testing recommended to confirm diagnosis
Nonclassic form:	• Controversial if nonclassic forms exist
Management:	• GC and MC replacement • Patients may need higher GC doses,[51] as hyperandrogenemia from accumulation of DHEAS can be difficult to control • Discussion regarding surgical correction of atypical genitalia • Sex hormones for patients who fail to progress through puberty (few)
11β-hydroxylase deficiency	
Prevalence:	• Second most common form of CAH (5%–8% of all cases) • 1:100,000; higher prevalence (15% of CAH) in Middle Eastern population[52]
Presentation:	• Adrenal insufficiency • 46,XX might have atypical genitalia and/or other signs of hyperandrogenism • Precocious puberty in both sexes • Low-renin hypertension due to excess DOC • Newborns can have mild, transient salt loss due to resistance to MC in infancy
Diagnosis:	• Excess 11-deoxycortisol and DOC • May be detected on newborn screening, as 17OHP might be sufficiently elevated
Nonclassic form:	• Rare[16]
Management:	• GC replacement at doses similar to 21OHD • Mineralocorticoid receptor antagonist
CYP17A1 deficiency (both 17α-hydroxylase deficiency and 17,20 lyase deficiency)	
Prevalence:	• 1:50,000; increased frequency in Brazil (second most common form after 21OHD)[53] due to presence of a founder mutation

(continued on next page)

Table 1 (continued)	
Presentation:	• Both gonads and adrenals affected • Impaired cortisol and sex steroid synthesis; aldosterone synthesis unaffected • Corticosterone excess compensates for cortisol deficiency • Excess DOC accumulation results in low-renin hypertension • Hypergonadotropic hypogonadism • 46,XX are normal at birth but may not undergo adrenarche or puberty • 46,XY have undervirilized external genitalia • Patients can have low bone mineral density even in absence of GC therapy[54]
Diagnosis:	• Elevated DOC, corticosterone, 18-OH-corticosterone and 18-OH-DOC and low concentrations of 17-hydroxylated steroids, which respond poorly to cosyntropin[15]
Nonclassic form:	• Not defined, although phenotypic variability occurs
Management:	• GC to suppress ACTH and excess mineralocorticoids • Age- and gender-appropriate sex-steroid replacement, if necessary
Isolated 17,20-lyase activity	
Prevalence:	• Extremely rare

Presentation:	• Can be caused by mutations in several different genes
	  ○ Specific mutations in the "redox partner-binding site" or the catalytic active site of CYP17A1
	  ○ Cytochrome b_5 (a protein that interacts with CYP17A1 to promote 17,20-lyase activity) deficiency leading to androgen deficiency with associated methemoglobinemia
	  ○ Rare mutations in the electron-donating domain of POR
	• Both gonads and adrenal glands affected
	• All reported patients so far are 46,XY likely due to ascertainment bias[50]

Diagnosis:	• Normal 17-hydroxycorticosteroids but markedly reduced sex steroids (DHEA, DHEAS, A4, T, DHT)
Nonclassic form:	• Not reported
Management:	• Age- and gender-appropriate sex-steroid replacement, if necessary
POR deficiency	
Prevalence:	• Incidence and phenotype vary with ethnicity but fairly common[15] • POR gene is highly polymorphic • Relatively newly recognized form of CAH, first described in 2004[55]

(continued on next page)

Table 1 (*continued*)	

Presentation:	• Characterized by partially deficient CYP17A1, with or without associated deficient activity of 21-hydroxylase and aromatase
	• Newborns often have associated skeletal defects called Antley-Bixler syndrome (ABS), characterized by craniosynostosis, radioulnar or radiohumeral synostosis, midface hypoplasia, and other skeletal manifestations. ABS may be seen in conditions other than CAH
	• Great variability in clinical and hormonal findings
	• Atypical genitalia in both sexes
	  ○ Incompletely developed external genitalia in affected boys due to defective testicular steroidogenesis
	  ○ Phenotype in girls varies with mutation; alternative "backdoor pathway" of androgen synthesis leads to excess synthesis of active androgens and results in atypical genitalia in 46,XX
	• Defective placental aromatase activity in some mutations permits fetal androgenic precursors to enter and virilize the mother during pregnancy, similar to women carrying a fetus with aromatase deficiency

Diagnosis:	• Near normal cortisol levels common, which respond poorly to cosyntropin • Usually have normal electrolytes and mineralocorticoid function • High concentration of 17OHP4 that responds variably to cosyntropin; some patients might be detected by newborn screening • Increased pregnenolone, progesterone, DOC, and corticosterone • Low levels of adrenal precursors of sex steroids like DHEA, A4 • Abnormal elevations of metabolites from "backdoor pathway"
Nonclassic form:	• Few patients diagnosed in newborn period
Management:	• Adrenal insufficiency present in most patients; cosyntropin test recommended for diagnosis[56] • Sex-hormone replacement at pubertal age

Abbreviations: 17OHP, 17α-hydroxyprogesterone; DOC, 11-deoxycorticosterone; GC, glucocorticoids; hCG, human chorionic gonadotropin; MC, mineralocorticoids; POR, P450 oxidoreductase; SCC, side chain cleavage; StAR, steroidogenic acute regulatory protein.
   Data from Refs.[15,16,50–56]

often present as adolescents or young adults with acne, hirsutism, menstrual abnormalities, or infertility, features that overlap greatly with those of polycystic ovarian syndrome (PCOS). Boys with NCCAH often remain undiagnosed, or only identified during genetic screening performed for preconception counseling or after the birth of an affected offspring.[5]

Female patients with nonclassic 3β-hydroxysteroid dehydrogenase type 2 (HSD3B2) or 11β-hydroxylase (CYP11B1) deficiency (11OHD) present with similar clinical features with those with 21OHD and PCOS, but both are extremely rare forms of CAH.[15,16] The distinction between these types of NCCAH and PCOS is unreliable based on clinical presentation alone.[17] Hirsutism (59% in NCCAH and 60%–70% in PCOS) and acne (33% in NCCAH and 14%–25% in PCOS) occur at comparable rates in both disorders.[18] In contrast, menstrual irregularity (10%–17% in women with NCCAH vs 75%–90% in PCOS)[18,19] and infertility (approximately 13% in NCCAH vs 25%–50% with PCOS) tend to occur more frequently among women with PCOS.[18] Similarly, polycystic ovarian morphology, although more common in PCOS, has also been reported in 30% to 40% patients with NCCAH.[18,19] Metabolic features typically associated with PCOS, including obesity, insulin resistance, and dyslipidemia, have also been reported in up to 40% of patients with NCCAH.[18,19] Although the prevalence of PCOS is about 40 to 50 times higher than that of nonclassic 21OHD among women with hyperandrogenemia,[18] testing for nonclassic 21OHD should be pursued in all such patients, as the correct diagnosis has implications for treatment and family planning.

BIOCHEMISTRY OF CONGENITAL ADRENAL HYPERPLASIA: IMPLICATION FOR DIAGNOSIS AND DISEASE MONITORING
Diagnosis of Congenital Adrenal Hyperplasia

All enzymatic defects within the steroidogenic pathway generate a large precursor to product ratio (see **Fig. 1**), which is further enhanced by ACTH stimulation. The prominent elevation of the main substrate for the defective enzyme forms the basis of CAH diagnosis. For 21OHD, the diagnosis relies on 17-hydroxyprogesterone (17OHP) elevations, which span a gradient reflective of the spectrum of enzymatic defects. Both neonatal and clinically prompted screening for 21OHD consists of 17OHP measurement, and values greater than 200 ng/dL (6 nmol/L) are suggestive of the diagnosis. Patients with classic 21OHD typically have 17OHP concentrations more than 10,000 ng/dL. In patients with modest 17OHP baseline elevations, of 200 to 1000 ng/dL (6–30 nmol/L), a cosyntropin stimulation test is the current standard of care, and 17OHP values greater than 1000 ng/dL establish the diagnosis.[2] Because 17OHP follows closely the circadian rhythm of ACTH, blood should be obtained in early morning. After puberty, 17OHP should be measured during the follicular phase to detect NCCAH, as ovarian surges of 17OHP occur during the luteal phase of the menstrual cycle.

A caveat to CAH testing is that these diagnostic thresholds should be considered in the context of the assay methodology, population, and individual background. Some patients with NCCAH could be missed based on a 17OHP cutoff greater than 200 ng/dL (>6 nmol/L),[20] and lower thresholds have been proposed, particularly when using mass spectrometry assays.[17,20,21] False positive 17OHP screening results are even more common, particularly when immunoassays are used, and when the blood sample is obtained in the luteal phase. Modestly elevated 17OHP is reported in 25% of women with PCOS,[19,22] likely because the high rates of irregular menses and amenorrhea make follicular phase testing impractical. Other tests suggestive of PCOS, such as elevated luteinizing hormone/follicle-stimulating hormone ratio, have poor sensitivity and specificity and can also be seen in approximately 10% women with NCCAH.[19] Simultaneous elevation of 21-deoxycortisol and lower corticosterone further support the diagnosis of CAH.[17,23] Such multi-steroid panels could circumvent the need for cosyntropin-stimulated testing in the future.

17OHP is typically elevated in patients with classic HSD3B2 deficiency or 11OHD,[1] although normal levels may be seen in nonclassic forms.[16] The diagnosis of nonclassic HSD3B2 deficiency is made when 17-hydroxypregnenolone exceeds 3000 ng/dL, along with a cortisol greater than 18 μg/dL after cosyntropin stimulation, and a 17-hydroxypregnenolone/cortisol ratio greater than 10 standard deviations above normal.[24] Nonclassic 11OHD is diagnosed when 11-deoxycortisol reaches concentrations greater than 1800 ng/dL and cortisol is greater than 18 µg/dL after cosyntropin.[25] Modestly abnormal baseline and even cosyntropin-stimulated steroid ratios can be deceiving, especially when immunoassays are used, and diagnostic confirmation with genetic testing is preferred for these very rare forms of CAH.

Androgen Excess in Congenital Adrenal Hyperplasia

Aside from its diagnostic significance, the excess 17OHP serves as substrate for fully functional enzymes, resulting in overproduction of adrenal androgens and precursors (see **Fig. 1**); this includes androstenedione (A4) and testosterone (T), as well as their 11-oxygenated metabolites, also called 11-oxyandrogens.[26] T and A4 are produced by both the gonads and adrenal glands, which might explain their poor correlation with clinical evidence of androgen excess in CAH patients.[27,28] In contrast, the major source of 11-oxyandrogens is the adrenal gland,[26] which expresses CYP11B1 abundantly.[29] In fact, 11-hydroxyandrostenedione (11OHA4) is the most abundant unconjugated C_{19} steroid produced by the healthy human adrenal gland,[30] and its synthesis is further enhanced in patients with classic[31] and nonclassic 21OHD.[23] The downstream metabolites of 11OHA4, 11-ketoandrostenedione (11KA4) and 11-ketotestosterone (11KT), are produced primarily in periphery.

In vitro studies have shown that 11KT is a bioactive androgen, with maximum androgen potency comparable with that of T.[32,33] Several lines of evidence also support the androgenic bioactivity of 11KT in vivo. 11KT has been associated with physiologic and premature adrenarche, and its concentrations exceed those of T before puberty.[32] 11-Oxyandrogens are 3- to 4-fold higher in patients with classic CAH relative to age- and sex-matched controls.[31] Higher concentrations of 11-oxyandrogens have been associated with higher adrenal volume, presence of testicular adrenal rest tumors, and menstrual irregularities in patients with classic CAH.[34] In addition, although in women with classic CAH, 11KT and T correlate directly, suggesting their common adrenal source, T correlates inversely with 11KT in sexually mature boys with classic 21OHD,[31] pointing toward hypothalamic-pituitary-gonadal axis suppression by excessive adrenal androgens in uncontrolled patients.

In a recent study of 86 patients undergoing testing for NCCAH, 11-oxyandrogens were disproportionately elevated relative to conventional androgens in patients with confirmed NCCAH versus those without CAH, 50% of whom had PCOS.[23] In contrast, A4 and T were similar between the 2 groups, reinforcing that the clinical utility of these traditional androgens in assessing the source of hyperandrogenism is limited. Generally, a high A4/T ratio is suggestive of adrenal androgen excess.[35] To further complicate things, however, women with CAH often secondarily develop PCOS,[36] and, conversely, a large subset of women with PCOS have increased adrenal androgen production.[37,38]

MANAGEMENT

The goal of treatment in patients with NCCAH is to suppress the excess adrenal androgen synthesis and the associated complications. Unlike patients with classic CAH, patients with NCCAH do not have adrenal insufficiency and do not need hormonal replacement with glucocorticoids. In children with precocious puberty or accelerated growth velocity, glucocorticoids may be used to suppress the ACTH-driven adrenal androgen excess.[2] Consideration for glucocorticoid discontinuation should be given once these children have attained their final adult height or 2 to 3 years after menarche for girls.[2]

For adolescents and adult women presenting with signs of hyperandrogenism, such as acne or hirsutism, oral contraceptive (OC) therapy with estrogen-progestin preparations is the treatment of choice.[39] Treatment with OCs reduces hyperandrogenemia by (a) suppression of luteinizing hormone and subsequently of ovarian androgen production; (b) stimulation of hepatic synthesis of sex hormone-binding globulin, with resultant reduction of free androgen concentration; (c) slight reduction of adrenal androgen synthesis; (d) decreased binding of androgens to their receptors; (e) increased clearance of T; and (f) mild inhibition in the pilosebaceous unit of 5α-reductase, the enzyme catalyzing conversion of T to the most potent androgen, dihydrotestosterone (DHT).[39] Although norgestimate is the only available progestin with low androgenicity that does not enhance the risk of venous thromboembolism compared to earlier generation progestins, evidence to support higher effectiveness of a particular OC for treating hirsutism is lacking. Women who present with hirsutism should be counseled about the expected timeframe for improvement, which may take as long as 6 to 12 months,[39] and the potential need for adjunct direct hair removal methods, like photoepilation or electrolysis.

Addition of antiandrogens can be considered if results are unsatisfactory with OCs alone. These therapies should never be used in reproductive-age women without reliable contraception methods, because of their potential effects on the developing male genitalia in utero. Spironolactone, primarily a mineralocorticoid antagonist, also has antiandrogenic effects.[40] Other therapies for hirsutism include finasteride, a 5α-reductase inhibitor, or cyproterone acetate, a progesterone derivative that competes with DHT for binding to androgen receptor (not available in the United States). Flutamide, a nonsteroidal androgen receptor blocker, is not recommended because of hepatotoxicity. Both spironolactone and finasteride have similar efficacy in improving hirsutism, with a pooled weighted mean difference of -7.02 (95% confidence interval [CI; -11.51 to -2.52]) Ferriman-Gallway units in comparison to placebo,[39,41] and their effect is additive to that of OCs, further reducing hirsutism pooled weighted Ferriman-Gallway units by -1.73 (95% CI [-3.32 to -0.13]).[41] Glucocorticoids are the mainstay of androgen suppression therapy only in classic CAH. Although glucocorticoids were shown to be more effective than OCs or antiandrogens for suppressing serum adrenal androgen concentrations in women with NCCAH, they were less effective in improving hirsutism,[42,43] with an increased risk of toxicity. Thus, glucocorticoids are only used for managing hirsutism in female patients with NCCAH when intolerance to OCs and/or antiandrogens has been established.[39]

Monitoring treatment of patients with NCCAH relies mostly on clinical evaluation, as reliable tests have been lacking. When elevated, T and A4 should be normalized, whereas 17OHP elevations should be permissible. Normalization of 17OHP typically indicates overtreatment with glucocorticoids. Interestingly, elevations of 11-oxyandrogens have been reported in a subset of women with PCOS relative to healthy controls.[44,45] Nevertheless, limited data suggest that these steroids might be higher in patients with NCCAH.[46] Although some commercial laboratories offer 11KT measurement, further studies are needed to clarify the clinical utility of 11-oxyandrogens as biomarkers of adrenal versus gonadal overactivity. Standardized protocols, with testing that accounts for circadian hormonal variations and that directly compares women with NCCAH and PCOS, will be essential to promulgate 11-oxyandrogens into future practical applications.

Pregnancy in Women with Nonclassic Congenital Adrenal Hyperplasia

For women with NCCAH with irregular or anovulatory cycles who are interested in conceiving, glucocorticoids are the first-line therapy.[47] Ovulation induction with clomiphene citrate, followed by other reproductive endocrinology interventions, is recommended when pregnancy is not achieved during treatment with glucocorticoids.[48]

Limited evidence suggests that treatment with glucocorticoids might reduce the time to conception and the risk of miscarriages in women with NCCAH, which occur at higher rates in this population as compared with healthy women.[2,11,12,49] Hydrocortisone, prednisone, and prednisolone are all safe to use in women attempting pregnancy, whereas dexamethasone, which is not inactivated by the placenta, should be avoided, because of risk of fetal hypothalamic-pituitary-adrenal axis and growth suppression.[2] Women with NCCAH who become pregnant spontaneously, without treatment with glucocorticoids, do not need to be treated with glucocorticoids.

Maternal 17OHP and A4 are elevated during pregnancy and cannot be used as biomarkers of CAH control. Hence, pregnant women should be followed clinically. Guidelines are lacking in regards to the optimal management of women with NCCAH during pregnancy. Some practices continue low doses of glucocorticoids throughout pregnancy if used preconception, whereas others stop glucocorticoids once pregnancy is confirmed or after the first trimester.

SUMMARY

NCCAH is a relatively common disease, and it should be suspected and excluded in all women with PCOS-like phenotype, including hirsutism, acne, and menstrual abnormalities. Other nonclassic forms of CAH that might mimic PCOS, such as HSD3B2 or CYP11B1 deficiencies, are extremely rare. Screening with 17OHP, followed by a confirmatory cosyntropin stimulation test if needed, establishes the diagnosis of 21OHD. Because hormonal cutoffs can be ambiguous, in part because of the low numbers, along with immunoassay artifacts, genetic testing is often indicated to confirm the very rare HSD3B2 or CYP11B1 deficiency when these forms of CAH are suspected based on clinical and hormonal abnormalities. Although the prevalence of PCOS far exceeds that of CAH, and although overlap in management exists (particularly for hirsutism and acne), treatment of infertility and preconception considerations warrant accurate diagnosis. Biomarkers indicative adrenal as opposed to gonadal androgen excess, such as 11-oxyandrogens, might facilitate the management of patients with hyperandrogenism; studies directly comparing patients with CAH and PCOS are lacking and will be key to translating pathophysiology knowledge into clinical applications.

CLINICS CARE POINTS

- Consider NCCAH in all patients with polycystic ovarian syndrome (PCOS)-like phenotype, as the two disorders have similar clinical presentation.
- Screening for NCCAH shodul be done by measuring 17α-hydroxyprogesterone (17OHP), ideally during the follicular phase (physiological elevations are possible during the luteal phase).
- When a screening 17OHP is elevated, NCCAH is confirmed or exlcuded with a cosyntropin stimulation test.
- Patients with NCCAH do not have adrenal insufficiency and do not need hormonal replacement.

- Glucocorticoids can be used in children with NCCAH who present with precocious puberty in order to suppress the adrenal androgen excess; the need for therapy should be reassessed after final height is attained.
- The treatment of women with NCCAH who present with signs of hyperandrogenism and who are not planning pregnancy is similar to those with PCOS, and includes oral contraceptives +/- anti-androgen therapy. Treatment of infertility, however, starts with glucocorticoids in NCCAH women.

ACKNOWLEDGMENTS

Fig. 1 was created using Biorender.com.

REFERENCES

1. Turcu AF, Auchus RJ. Adrenal steroidogenesis and congenital adrenal hyperplasia. Endocrinol Metab Clin North Am 2015;44(2):275–96.
2. Speiser PW, Arlt W, Auchus RJ, et al. Congenital adrenal hyperplasia due to steroid 21-hydroxylase deficiency: an Endocrine Society Clinical Practice Guideline. J Clin Endocrinol Metab 2018;103(11):4043–88.
3. Hannah-Shmouni F, Morissette R, Sinaii N, et al. Revisiting the prevalence of nonclassic congenital adrenal hyperplasia in US Ashkenazi Jews and Caucasians. Genet Med 2017;19(11):1276–9.
4. Speiser PW, Dupont B, Rubinstein P, et al. High frequency of nonclassical steroid 21-hydroxylase deficiency. Am J Hum Genet 1985;37(4):650–67.
5. Carmina E, Dewailly D, Escobar-Morreale HF, et al. Non-classic congenital adrenal hyperplasia due to 21-hydroxylase deficiency revisited: an update with a special focus on adolescent and adult women. Hum Reprod Update 2017;23(5):580–99.
6. Carroll MC, Campbell RD, Porter RR. Mapping of steroid 21-hydroxylase genes adjacent to complement component C4 genes in HLA, the major histocompatibility complex in man. Proc Natl Acad Sci U S A 1985;82(2):521–5.
7. White PC, Grossberger D, Onufer BJ, et al. Two genes encoding steroid 21-hydroxylase are located near the genes encoding the fourth component of complement in man. Proc Natl Acad Sci U S A 1985;82(4):1089–93.
8. White PC, New MI, Dupont B. Structure of human steroid 21-hydroxylase genes. Proc Natl Acad Sci U S A 1986;83(14):5111–5.
9. Miller WL, Merke DP. Tenascin-X, congenital adrenal hyperplasia, and the CAH-X syndrome. Horm Res paediatrics 2018;89(5):352–61.
10. White PC, Speiser PW. Congenital adrenal hyperplasia due to 21-hydroxylase deficiency. Endocr Rev 2000;21(3):245–91.
11. Moran C, Azziz R, Weintrob N, et al. Reproductive outcome of women with 21-hydroxylase-deficient nonclassic adrenal hyperplasia. J Clin Endocrinol Metab 2006;91(9):3451–6.
12. Bidet M, Bellanne-Chantelot C, Galand-Portier MB, et al. Fertility in women with nonclassical congenital adrenal hyperplasia due to 21-hydroxylase deficiency. J Clin Endocrinol Metab 2010;95(3):1182–90.
13. New MI, Abraham M, Gonzalez B, et al. Genotype-phenotype correlation in 1,507 families with congenital adrenal hyperplasia owing to 21-hydroxylase deficiency. Proc Natl Acad Sci U S A 2013;110(7):2611–6.
14. Finkielstain GP, Chen W, Mehta SP, et al. Comprehensive genetic analysis of 182 unrelated families with congenital adrenal hyperplasia due to 21-hydroxylase deficiency. J Clin Endocrinol Metab 2011;96(1):E161–72.

15. Miller WL, Auchus RJ. The molecular biology, biochemistry, and physiology of human steroidogenesis and its disorders. Endocr Rev 2011;32(1):81–151.
16. Reisch N, Hogler W, Parajes S, et al. A diagnosis not to be missed: nonclassic steroid 11beta-hydroxylase deficiency presenting with premature adrenarche and hirsutism. J Clin Endocrinol Metab 2013;98(10):E1620–5.
17. Oriolo C, Fanelli F, Castelli S, et al. Steroid biomarkers for identifying non-classic adrenal hyperplasia due to 21-hydroxylase deficiency in a population of PCOS with suspicious levels of 17OH-progesterone. J Endocrinol Invest 2020;43(10): 1499–509.
18. Papadakis G, Kandaraki EA, Tseniklidi E, et al. Polycystic ovary syndrome and NC-CAH: distinct characteristics and common findings. a systematic review. Front Endocrinol (Lausanne) 2019;10:388.
19. Pall M, Azziz R, Beires J, et al. The phenotype of hirsute women: a comparison of polycystic ovary syndrome and 21-hydroxylase-deficient nonclassic adrenal hyperplasia. Fertil Steril 2010;94(2):684–9.
20. Maffazioli GDN, Bachega T, Hayashida SAY, et al. Steroid screening tools differentiating nonclassical congenital adrenal hyperplasia and polycystic ovary syndrome. J Clin Endocrinol Metab 2020;105(8):dgaa369.
21. Escobar-Morreale HF, Sanchon R, San Millan JL. A prospective study of the prevalence of nonclassical congenital adrenal hyperplasia among women presenting with hyperandrogenic symptoms and signs. J Clin Endocrinol Metab 2008;93(2): 527–33.
22. Rudnicka E, Kunicki M, Radowicki S. [Androgen and 17-hydroxyprogesterone concentrations in blood serum versus menstrual patterns in women with polycystic ovary syndrome (PCOS)]. Ginekol Pol 2010;81(10):745–9.
23. Turcu AF, El-Maouche D, Zhao L, et al. Androgen excess and diagnostic steroid biomarkers for nonclassic 21-hydroxylase deficiency without cosyntropin stimulation. Eur J Endocrinol 2020;183(1):63–71.
24. Mermejo LM, Elias LL, Marui S, et al. Refining hormonal diagnosis of type II 3β-hydroxysteroid dehydrogenase deficiency in patients with premature pubarche and hirsutism based on HSD3B2 genotyping. J Clin Endocrinol Metab 2005;90(3): 1287–93.
25. White PC, Curnow KM, Pascoe L. Disorders of steroid 11β-hydroxylase isozymes. Endocr Rev 1994;15(4):421–38.
26. Turcu AF, Rege J, Auchus RJ, et al. 11-Oxygenated androgens in health and disease. Nat Rev Endocrinol 2020;16(5):284–96.
27. Speiser PW, Dupont J, Zhu D, et al. Disease expression and molecular genotype in congenital adrenal hyperplasia due to 21-hydroxylase deficiency. J Clin Invest 1992;90(2):584–95.
28. Krone N, Braun A, Roscher AA, et al. Predicting phenotype in steroid 21-hydroxylase deficiency? Comprehensive genotyping in 155 unrelated, well defined patients from southern Germany. J Clin Endocrinol Metab 2000;85(3):1059–65.
29. Rege J, Nakamura Y, Wang T, et al. Transcriptome profiling reveals differentially expressed transcripts between the human adrenal zona fasciculata and zona reticularis. J Clin Endocrinol Metab 2014;99(3):E518–27.
30. Rege J, Nakamura Y, Satoh F, et al. Liquid chromatography-tandem mass spectrometry analysis of human adrenal vein 19-carbon steroids before and after ACTH stimulation. J Clin Endocrinol Metab 2013;98(3):1182–8.
31. Turcu AF, Nanba AT, Chomic R, et al. Adrenal-derived 11-oxygenated 19-carbon steroids are the dominant androgens in classic 21-hydroxylase deficiency. Eur J Endocrinol 2016;174(5):601–9.

32. Rege J, Turcu AF, Kasa-Vubu JZ, et al. 11-ketotestosterone is the dominant circulating bioactive androgen during normal and premature adrenarche. J Clin Endocrinol Metab 2018;103(12):4589–98.

33. Pretorius E, Africander DJ, Vlok M, et al. 11-ketotestosterone and 11-ketodihydrotestosterone in castration resistant prostate cancer: potent androgens which can no longer be ignored. PloS one 2016;11(7):e0159867.

34. Turcu AF, Mallappa A, Elman MS, et al. 11-Oxygenated androgens are biomarkers of adrenal volume and testicular adrenal rest tumors in 21-hydroxylase deficiency. J Clin Endocrinol Metab 2017;102(8):2701–10.

35. Auchus RJ, Arlt W. Approach to the patient: the adult with congenital adrenal hyperplasia. J Clin Endocrinol Metab 2013;98(7):2645–55.

36. Barnes RB, Rosenfield RL, Ehrmann DA, et al. Ovarian hyperandrogynism as a result of congenital adrenal virilizing disorders: evidence for perinatal masculinization of neuroendocrine function in women. J Clin Endocrinol Metab 1994;79(5):1328–33.

37. Azziz R, Black V, Hines GA, et al. Adrenal androgen excess in the polycystic ovary syndrome: sensitivity and responsivity of the hypothalamic-pituitary-adrenal axis. J Clin Endocrinol Metab 1998;83(7):2317–23.

38. Puurunen J, Piltonen T, Jaakkola P, et al. Adrenal androgen production capacity remains high up to menopause in women with polycystic ovary syndrome. J Clin Endocrinol Metab 2009;94(6):1973–8.

39. Martin KA, Anderson RR, Chang RJ, et al. Evaluation and treatment of hirsutism in premenopausal women: an Endocrine Society Clinical Practice Guideline. J Clin Endocrinol Metab 2018;103(4):1233–57.

40. Corvol P, Michaud A, Menard J, et al. Antiandrogenic effect of spirolactones: mechanism of action. Endocrinology 1975;97(1):52–8.

41. Swiglo BA, Cosma M, Flynn DN, et al. Clinical review: antiandrogens for the treatment of hirsutism: a systematic review and metaanalyses of randomized controlled trials. J Clin Endocrinol Metab 2008;93(4):1153–60.

42. Frank-Raue K, Junga G, Raue F, et al. Therapy of hirsutism in females with adrenal enzyme defects of steroid hormone biosynthesis: comparison of dexamethasone with cyproterone acetate. Klin Wochenschr 1990;68(12):597–601.

43. Spritzer P, Billaud L, Thalabard JC, et al. Cyproterone acetate versus hydrocortisone treatment in late-onset adrenal hyperplasia. J Clin Endocrinol Metab 1990;70(3):642–6.

44. O'Reilly MW, Kempegowda P, Jenkinson C, et al. 11-Oxygenated C19 steroids are the predominant androgens in polycystic ovary syndrome. J Clin Endocrinol Metab 2016;102(3):840–8.

45. Yoshida T, Matsuzaki T, Miyado M, et al. 11-Oxygenated C19 steroids as circulating androgens in women with polycystic ovary syndrome. Endocr J 2018;65(10):979–90.

46. Turcu AF, Wannachalee T, Tsodikov A, et al. Comprehensive analysis of steroid biomarkers for guiding primary aldosteronism subtyping. Hypertension 2020;75(1):183–92.

47. Birnbaum MD, Rose LI. The partial adrenocortical hydroxylase deficiency syndrome in infertile women. Fertil steril 1979;32(5):536–41.

48. Lo JC, Grumbach MM. Pregnancy outcomes in women with congenital virilizing adrenal hyperplasia. Endocrinol Metab Clin North Am 2001;30(1):207–29.

49. Eyal O, Ayalon-Dangur I, Segev-Becker A, et al. Pregnancy in women with nonclassic congenital adrenal hyperplasia: time to conceive and outcome. Clin Endocrinol (Oxf) 2017;87(5):552–6.

50. Miller WL. Mechanisms in endocrinology: rare defects in adrenal steroidogenesis. Eur J Endocrinol 2018;179(3):R125–41.
51. Al Alawi AM, Nordenstrom A, Falhammar H. Clinical perspectives in congenital adrenal hyperplasia due to 3beta-hydroxysteroid dehydrogenase type 2 deficiency. Endocrine 2019;63(3):407–21.
52. Khattab A, Haider S, Kumar A, et al. Clinical, genetic, and structural basis of congenital adrenal hyperplasia due to 11beta-hydroxylase deficiency. Proc Natl Acad Sci U S A 2017;114(10):E1933–40.
53. Costa-Santos M, Kater CE, Auchus RJ. Brazilian congenital adrenal hyperplasia multicenter study G. Two prevalent CYP17 mutations and genotype-phenotype correlations in 24 Brazilian patients with 17-hydroxylase deficiency. J Clin Endocrinol Metab 2004;89(1):49–60.
54. Sousa Paredes SC, Marques O, Alves M. Partial deficiency of 17alpha-hydroxylase: a rare cause of congenital adrenal hyperplasia. BMJ Case Rep 2019;12(12).
55. Arlt W, Walker EA, Draper N, et al. Congenital adrenal hyperplasia caused by mutant P450 oxidoreductase and human androgen synthesis: analytical study. Lancet 2004;363(9427):2128–35.
56. Krone N, Reisch N, Idkowiak J, et al. Genotype-phenotype analysis in congenital adrenal hyperplasia due to P450 oxidoreductase deficiency. J Clin Endocrinol Metab 2012;97(2):E257–67.

Moving?

Make sure your subscription moves with you!

To notify us of your new address, find your **Clinics Account Number** (located on your mailing label above your name), and contact customer service at:

Email: journalscustomerservice-usa@elsevier.com

800-654-2452 (subscribers in the U.S. & Canada)
314-447-8871 (subscribers outside of the U.S. & Canada)

Fax number: 314-447-8029

Elsevier Health Sciences Division
Subscription Customer Service
3251 Riverport Lane
Maryland Heights, MO 63043

*To ensure uninterrupted delivery of your subscription, please notify us at least 4 weeks in advance of move.